Micro-Immunotherapy

Diagnostics and Therapy of Immunological Diseases

Corinne I. Heitz, PhD

ML VERLAG

Important note: The statements made in this book regarding methods, risks, etc., have been meticulously compiled and verified by the author. However, all information is presented without any guarantee. Neither the author nor the publisher can be held liable for any disadvantages or damages that may result from the advice provided in this book. The guidance offered in this book cannot and is not intended to substitute for professional advice from a doctor or healthcare practitioner.

1st Edition 2024

kontakt@mgo-fachverlage.de

Proofreading: Matt Corby-Eaglen

Printed by: Generál Nyomda Kft., H-6727 Szeged

Picture credits
Cover photo: Fotolia.de – bluebay2014, freshidea, fotoliaxrender; Corinne I. Heitz
others: Fotolia.de – freshidea, fotoliaxrender, angellodeco, psdesign1; Corinne I. Heitz

www.ml-buchverlag.de

ISBN (book): 978-3-96474-732-7
ISBN (E-Book/PDF): 978-3-96474-733-4

Table of Contents

Preface to the First Edition in English by the Author

I am delighted to present this book to my colleagues who do not speak German. The book "Mikroimmuntherapie" was originally published in 2011. The version you are holding is the translation of the third revised edition, published in 2021.

This book represents the first English edition and covers the fundamental knowledge of Micro-Immunotherapy. However, it is essential to note that the field of immunology is constantly evolving, and new research findings continuously update our understanding of cytokines and information on pathogens. As a result, this book may not be exhaustive, and I make no claim to absolute completeness.

Throughout my work, I have aimed not to disassemble and analyse everything in isolation but to discover the synthesis of interconnected elements. The immune system, in particular, serves as a remarkable example of interconnectedness and forms an intricate network. My training and practical experience have taught me to approach the complexity of the immune system with humility and utmost respect.

I am fully aware that the Ultima Ratio – the final conclusion – may remain elusive and may never be fully attained. Within the immune system, I perceive something akin to a "divine plan," or for those preferring a scientific perspective, a genius plan of creation that bestows uniqueness on each individual through genetics and the immune system.

The immune system is a remarkable system within our body. In my opinion, the notion that the immune system functions incorrectly and causes aggressive autoimmune diseases is not accurate. Suppressing the immune system or certain parts of it cannot be the right approach. The immune system performs its task efficiently, but there may be underlying causes (often viral reactivations) that lead to an abnormal immune response. Identifying these causes is a key aspect of Micro-Immunotherapy, known as diagnostics.

Micro-Immunotherapy treatment relies on immunological knowledge, utilizing the immune system itself to "heal" diseases. Healing is achievable because the human body is dynamic. The immune system eliminates damaged cells while healthy cells multiply, eventually resulting in more healthy cells than sick ones. This leads to a path of self-healing, which is why this form of therapy may take longer.

Today, Micro-Immunotherapy has become an established therapeutic concept that employs carefully selected combinations of diluted cytokines. It aims to modulate and harmonize the intricate network of the immune system without causing any negative impact, which is often seen with allopathic agents such as interferon[1], corticoids[2], or cytostatics[3].

One of the notable advantages of this therapy is that it adheres to the dilution principles of homeopathy, ensuring that there are no toxic burdens or undesirable side effects associated with its use.

Similar to the application of homeopathic remedies, Micro-Immunotherapy may initially lead to a temporary worsening of symptoms. However, it does not result in the development of new perceptible illnesses or measurable disturbances of the immune system.

1 Interferons play a significant role in immunotherapy, with distinct types such as alpha, beta, and gamma interferons. Beta interferons are primarily utilized in the treatment of autoimmune diseases, particularly multiple sclerosis.

2 Corticoids find application in the treatment of various conditions such as asthma, autoimmune diseases, cluster headaches, eczema, epilepsy, acute hearing loss, acute tinnitus, nephritis, neurodermatitis, and specific chemotherapies for Hodgkin's disease and non-Hodgkin's lymphoma. They possess immunosuppressive properties, meaning they inhibit and weaken the immune system.

3 Cytostatic drugs disrupt metabolic processes associated with cell growth and division. As a result, they primarily target rapidly dividing cells, including hair follicle cells and mucosal epithelium in the mouth and gastrointestinal tract. Tumor cells, which have an increased rate of cell division and limited repair capacity, are more sensitive to cytostatic drugs compared to healthy cells. It is this difference that enables therapy with these highly toxic substances.

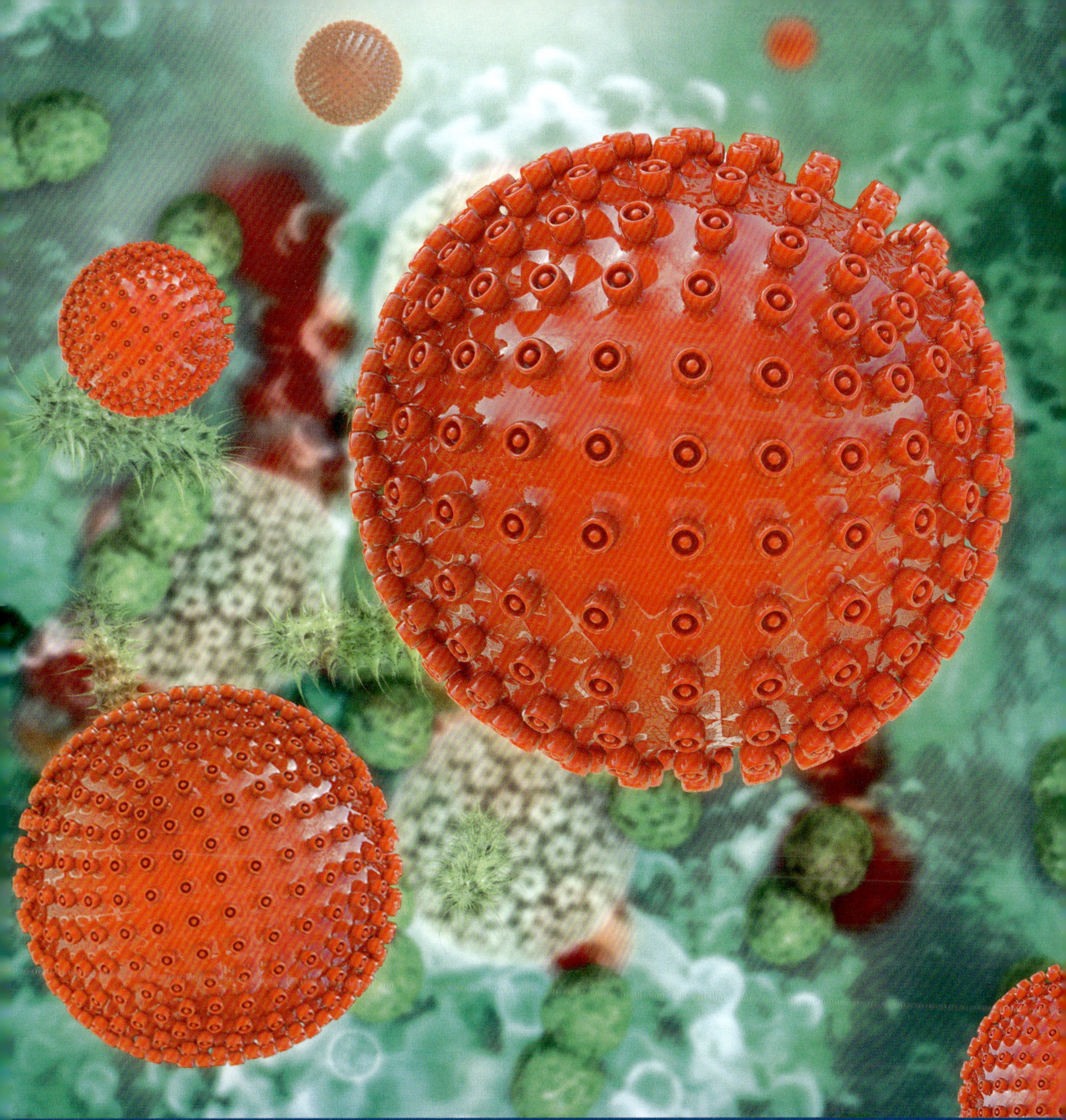

Theoretical Part

The theoretical part provides a simplified explanation of how the immune system functions and introduces the concepts of analytics for Micro-Immunotherapy and the theory of therapy.

In the subsequent practical part, the step-by-step interpretation of the analysis and the corresponding therapy are explained.

To understand and interpret the analytics (special blood tests), it is necessary to acquire some basic knowledge of immunology.

Although the workings of the immune system are highly complex, the evaluation and determination of the appropriate therapy can be simplified by following the basic guidelines described.

Micro-Immunotherapy focuses on identifying the causes and triggers of diseases. It operates under the assumption that chronic diseases are associated with pathogens, such as viruses, bacteria, or parasites, which burden our immune system and lead to illness. Alternatively, immune system dysregulation, either weakened or overreactive, can also contribute to the development of diseases.

Another area of interest in Micro-Immunotherapy is the treatment of various types of cancer, including solid tumours and leukaemia (blood cancer).

In essence, the following factors are examined during the analysis:

- Triggers (pathogens)
- State of the immune system
- And, where applicable, the genetic predisposition

In response to popular demand, a list of individual pathogens and their corresponding symptoms is provided. However, it is important to note that not every patient experiences the same symptoms, and the manifestation of symptoms can vary.

1 Viruses

The primary triggers are viruses, although bacteria can also be involved but less frequently. The focus is typically on viral reactivations or initial infections, especially those pathogens that integrate their genetic material into the host's DNA, making them capable of reactivation or persistence. DNA viruses, in particular, have the ability to influence cellular processes during division, leading to chronic diseases and potentially cancer.

DNA viruses are classified into five families.

1.1 Herpesvirus Family

Herpesviridae, named after the Greek word "herpes" meaning "to crawl," are enveloped, double-stranded DNA viruses characterized by an icosahedral capsid (a protein envelope consisting of triangular surfaces) surrounded by an envelope membrane. While herpes viruses are often associated with HSV-1 and HSV-2, the herpes virus group encompasses eight different human pathogenic herpes viruses (HHV) divided into three groups.

Alpha-Herpesviruses

... reproduce rapidly, have a wide host range, and establish lifelong infections in the host's ganglia:

- *HHV-1: Herpes Simplex Virus Type 1 (HSV-1)*
- *HHV-2: Herpes Simplex Virus Type 2 (HSV-2)*

Symptoms and clinical manifestations include:

- Herpes labialis (cold sores)
- Genital herpes
- Bell's palsy
- Trigeminal neuralgia
- Stomatitis aphthosa
- Prostatitis
- Urethritis
- Cervical changes
- Possible association with abortions
- Tendency to form cysts
- Endometriosis may also be linked to Herpes viruses types 1 or 2

Reactivations of alpha herpesviruses are often observed in chronic inflammation of the digestive tract with positive IgA.

From personal experience, they are frequently involved in tinnitus and neurodermatitis.

▸ *HHV-3: Varicella-Zoster Virus (VZV)*

Disease patterns include:

- Chickenpox
- Reactivation leading to shingles (herpes zoster)
- Zoster ophthalmicus affecting the face and eyes, which can cause corneal scarring and partial or complete blindness. Facial nerves may be affected, resulting in temporary paralysis (facial paresis) or loss of taste sensation.
- Zoster oticus affecting the auditory canal and/or auricle. Along with the severe pain associated with zoster, it can lead to hearing difficulties (cochlear nerve) and balance disturbances (vestibular nerve). Consider herpes zoster in cases of tinnitus.
- Zoster generalisatus, a systemic involvement of the entire nervous system, which is life-threatening but usually occurs in individuals with weakened immune systems (e.g., AIDS, leukaemia, or other forms of cancer).
- Zoster genitalis occurring in the genital area, accompanied by lymphatic swellings.
- Zoster disseminatus when the viruses spread through the bloodstream.
- Zoster meningitis, encephalitis, and myelitis.

Beta-Herpesviruses

... reproduce slowly and have a limited host range:

▸ *HHV-5: Cytomegalovirus (CMV), causing cytomegaly.*

Disease patterns include:

- Initial infection is usually asymptomatic.
- Rarely, symptoms may resemble flu, including fever, liver swelling, muscle pain, and body aches.
- CMV infections during pregnancy can cause severe damage to the central nervous system and brain in new-borns.

- Immunocompromised individuals may experience the following serious complications:
  - Retinitis (CMV retinitis)
  - Oesophagitis, enteritis
  - Pneumonia (CMV pneumonia)
  - Encephalitis (CMV encephalitis)
  - Cholangitis

▶ *HHV-6: Human Herpes Virus 6*

Disease patterns include:
- Three-day fever
- There is ongoing discussion regarding its potential connection to multiple sclerosis[4] and encephalopathies (inflammatory lesions).
- Chronic fatigue syndrome (CFS)

▶ *HHV-7: Human Herpes Virus 7*

Disease patterns include:
- Three-day fever
- Pityriasis rosea (rose lichen)
- Neurological diseases

Gamma Herpesviruses

... have varying replication times and a limited host range:

▶ *HHV-4: Epstein-Barr Virus (EBV)*

Disease patterns include:
- Mononucleosis
- EBV-associated diseases and symptoms (refer to page 50 for more details).

4 Latham LB, Lee MJ, Lincoln JA, Ji N, Forsthuber TG, Lindsey JW: Antiviral immune activity in multiple sclerosis cor- relates with MRI activity. Acta Neurol Scand. 2015 May 4. doi: 10.1111/ane.124 17. http://www.ncbi.nlm.nih.gov/ pubmed/25939660 [retrieved: 14 May 2015].

▸ *HHV-8: Human Herpes Virus 8*

Disease patterns include:

- Kaposi's sarcoma
- Certain lymphomas
- There is ongoing discussion regarding its potential connection to essential hypertension.

1.2 Papovaviridae

- Papillomaviruses, such as HPV
- Polyomaviridae, e.g., Simian virus 40[5]

1.3 Adenoviridae

Adenoviruses are typically common pathogens responsible for acute respiratory diseases. They are not considered the causative agents of chronic diseases[6].

1.4 Hepatitis Viruses

- Hepatitis A
- Hepatitis B
- Hepatitis C
- Hepatitis D and E

Hepatitis viruses include both DNA and RNA viruses. For example, hepatitis B and C are DNA viruses.

5 Simian virus 40 (SV-40), a virus belonging to the Polyomaviridae family and the genus Polyomavirus, is known for its role in the development of cancer cells through its oncogenes. An interesting and concerning fact is that SV-40 was discovered in kidney cell cultures from rhesus monkeys that were utilized in the production of polio vaccines. Between 1955 and 1963, it is estimated that millions of individuals received oral and injectable polio vaccines, potentially resulting in SV-40 infection.
Martini F. et al: Simian virus 40 in humans, Infectious Agents and Cancer20072:13 DOI: 10.1186/1750-9378-2-13 © Martini et al; licensee BioMed Central Ltd. 2007 [retrieved: 3/16/2021].

6 Human adenoviruses are a group of pathogenic viruses that belong to the Adenoviridae family and the Mastadenovirus genus. They were initially discovered in human adenoids, which is how they derived their name. Adenoviruses primarily cause respiratory tract illnesses. However, depending on the specific serotype, they can also be responsible for various other diseases, particularly in individuals with weakened immune systems. Additionally, there has been speculation about a potential link between Ad-36 type adenovirus and obesity.

2 Bacteria

There are several intracellular bacteria that can also lead to chronic and persistent diseases. The list is in alphabetical order and independent of pathogenicity.

2.1 Bartonella

Bartonella, including Bartonella quintana and Bartonella henselae, is responsible for several diseases. Bartonella quintana causes a condition known as five-day fever (Wolhynian fever).

▶ *Bartonella Henselae*

Bartonella henselae, commonly transmitted through cat scratches (zoonosis), causes cat scratch disease, which is typically a benign and self-limiting infection. It primarily leads to enlargement of axillary or cervical lymph nodes.

While most cases of cat scratch disease resolve without complications, there are potential complications such as:

- high fever,
- limb pain,
- headaches,
- and involvement of the nervous system (encephalitis, paralysis, neuroretinitis, radiculitis, polyneuritis).
- Systemic spread of skin papules,
- osteomyelitis,
- pneumonia,
- haemolysis,
- thrombocytopenia,
- and endocarditis are also observed in some cases.

2.2 Borrelia

Borrelia bacteria, including Borrelia burgdorferi and Borrelia recurrentis, are associated with various diseases:

▶ *Borrelia Burgdorferi*

Borrelia burgdorferi gained recognition in 1982 when it was identified as the pathogen responsible for tick-borne Lyme disease. Typical symptoms of Lyme disease

Include:

- headache,
- erythema migrans,
- erythema chronicum migrans,
- neurological symptoms,
- Garin-Bujadoux-Bannwarth syndrome (meningopolyneuritis GBB),
- arthritis,
- acrodermatitis chronica atrophicans,
- carditis,
- and eye involvement.

▶ *Borrelia Recurrentis*

Borrelia recurrentis causeslouse fever, transmitted by clothes lice. It is prevalent in cooler regions of Africa, South America, and Asia, and presents with severe fever attacks. Regional variations of Borrelia bacteria can trigger diseases like relapsing fever.

2.3 Chlamydia

Chlamydia comprises several species, including Chlamydia psittaci and Chlamydia trachomatis:

▶ *Chlamydia Psittaci*

Chlamydia psittaci is responsible for ornithosis, a disease transmitted by birds (zoonosis).

Psittacosis, also known as parrot disease, predominantly affects the lungs and manifests as a severe flu-like illness. The pathogen is primarily derived from birds such as parrots, parakeets, and pigeons, which often show no or minimal symptoms. The disease, previously known as pigeon fancier's disease, is recognized as an occupational hazard.

▶ *Chlamydia Trachomatis*

Chlamydia trachomatis is the most common bacterial cause of sexually transmitted infections in Europe. It leads to various symptoms, including pain during urination and swimming pool conjunctivitis[7].

7 Conjunctivitis of the eye typically after swimming in the pool

▶ *Yersinia Enterocolitica and Yersinia Pseudotuberculosis*

... responsible for febrile intestinal inflammations (enterocolitis or enteritis) resulting from food infection. These bacteria are associated with yersiniosis.

Common symptoms of Yersinia infections include

- recurring abdominal cramps with diarrhea,
- irritable bowel,
- pseudo-Crohn's disease,
- terminal ileitis,
- erythema nodosum,
- reactive Yersinia arthritis, and Reiter's disease with eczema of the palms and soles [10].

The clinical finding of mesenteric lymphadenitis[11], often difficult to distinguish from appendicitis, is also referred to as "pseudoappendicitis."

Yersinia species produce proteins released into the environment, known as "YOPs" (Yersinia outer proteins). These proteins possess pathogenic properties, interfering with phagocytosis as part of the immune defense mechanism.

Certain pathogenic Yersinia species produce siderophores[12], low-molecular compounds that facilitate iron supply through iron (III) ions. One well-known siderophore is yersiniabactin (Ybt)[13], found in Y. pestis, Y. pseudotuberculosis, and some strains of Y. enterocolitica.

---

10 Kato Y., Hattori T., Oh-Ya H., Yoshino S., Kato H.: Acute terminal ileitis and Yersinia enterocolitica infection. Gastroenterol Jpn. 1977;12(1):36-43. http://www.ncbi.nlm.nih.gov/pubmed/863177 [accessed 16 Mar 2021].

11 In mesenteric lymphadenitis (also known as mesenteric pseudoappendicitis), the lymph nodes in the ileocecal region become swollen due to inflammation of the ileum (ileitis). This condition is commonly observed as a result of viral systemic infections caused by adenoviruses, Epstein-Barr virus, cytomegalovirus, or rotaviruses. Nonspecific mesenteric lymphadenitis frequently coexists with these viral infections.

12 From the Greek: Iron bearer

13 Chaturvedi ,KS., Hung CS., Crowley JR., Stapleton AE., Henderson JP.: The siderophore yersiniabactin binds copper to protect pathogens during infection.

3 Parasites

3.1 Toxoplasma Gondii

Toxoplasmosis is a prevalent infectious disease primarily associated with cats. The causative agent of this disease is the parasite Toxoplasma gondii. In healthy individuals with a competent immune system, the infection often remains asymptomatic.

Symptoms, when present, can resemble those of a flu-like illness and may include:

- Mild fever
- Swollen lymph nodes in the neck
- Fatigue
- Headache and limb pain

Complications may arise in individuals with weakened immune systems, and these can manifest as:

- Inflammatory lesions, particularly in the brain
- Meningitis
- Changes in personality
- Paralysis and seizures
- Pneumonia

If a pregnant woman acquires an initial infection during the first or second trimester, it can lead to significant harm to the unborn child[14].

Recent studies have suggested potential connections between Toxoplasma infection and schizophrenia[15] in humans. Furthermore, there seems to be an association between latent toxoplasmosis and suicidal behavior[16].

For more in-depth information on additional pathogens and their pathological properties, please refer to "Praxisbuch Mikroimmuntherapie", 1st edition 2022, ISBN 978-3-96474-243-8 (in German).

---

14 Nat Chem Biol. 2012 Aug;8(8):731-6. doi: 10.1038/nchembio.1020. Epub 2012 Jul 8. http://www.ncbi.nlm.nih.gov/pubmed/22772152 [retrieved 16.3.2021]

15 Wang H-L et al: Prevalence of Toxoplasma infection in first-episode schizophrenia and comparison between Toxoplasma-seropositive and Toxoplasma-seronegative schizophrenia. Acta Psychiatrica Scandinavica 2006; 114: 40-48.

16 Y. Zhang, L. Träskman-Bendz, S. Janelidze, P. Langenberg, A. Saleh, N. Constantine, O. Okusaga, C. Bay-Richter, L. Brundin, T. T. Postolache: Toxoplasma gondii immunoglobulin G antibodies and nonfatal suicidal self-directed violence. In: The Journal of clinical psychiatry. Volume 73, Number 8, August 2012, pp. 1069-1076, http://www.ncbi.nlm.nih.gov/pubmed/22938818 [accessed 16.3.2021].

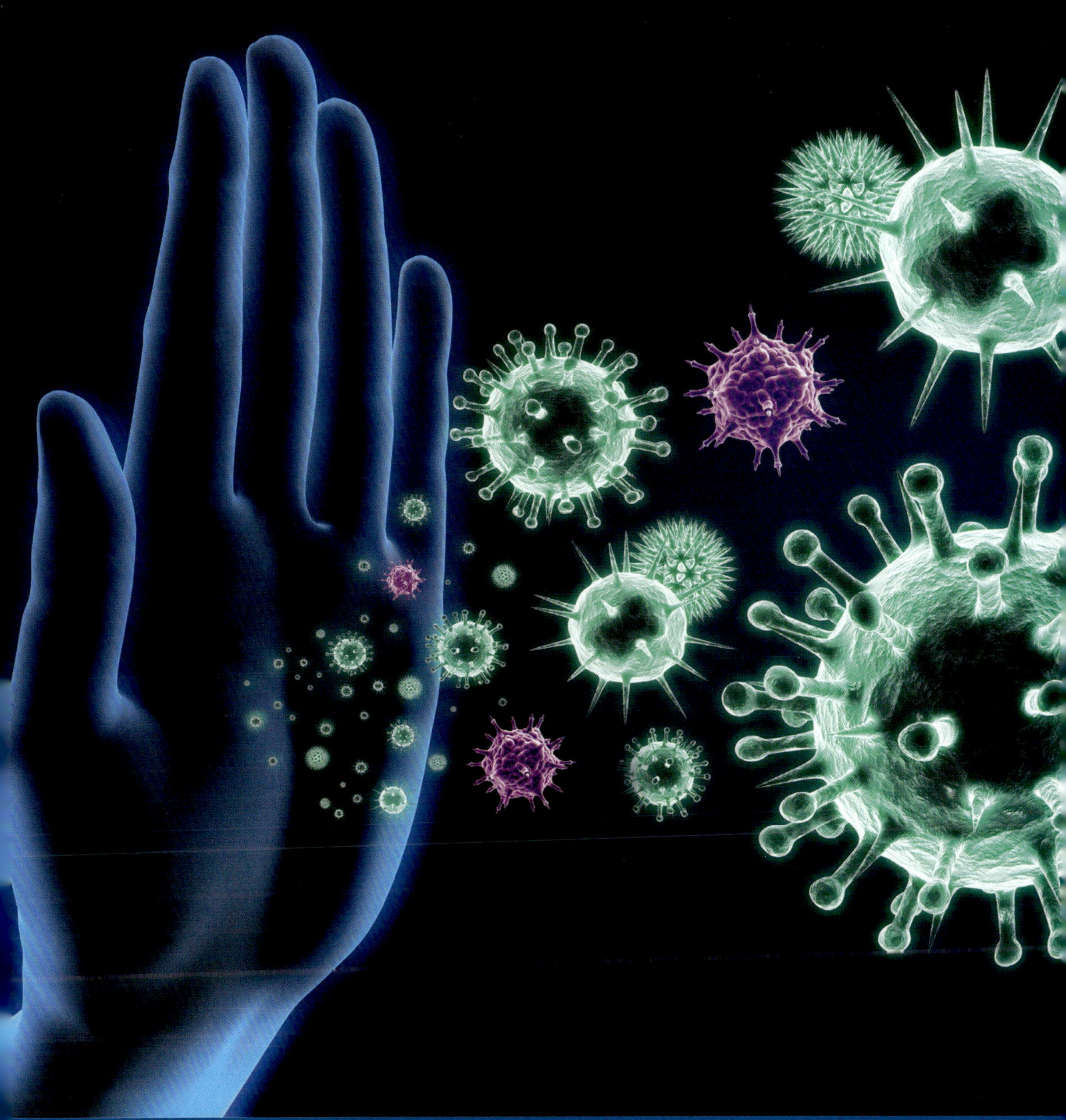

The Functioning of the Immune System

4 Brief Introduction to the Immune System

4.1 Origin of the Immune Cells

Immune cells are derived from a common stem cell that possesses two fundamental properties. Firstly, it has the ability to self-renew and sustain itself as a stem cell. Secondly, it has the capacity to differentiate into various types of cells with distinct properties.

The process of differentiation occurs through three primary pathways:

1. The hematopoietic stem cell gives rise to the myeloid progenitor cell, the lymphoid progenitor cell, and the null cell.
2. The myeloid progenitor cell further differentiates into cells responsible for nonspecific immune defense, such as monocytes, macrophages, and granulocytes.
3. The lymphoid precursor cell generates cells involved in specific immune defense. These cells form the lymphatic defense system, including B and T lymphocytes.

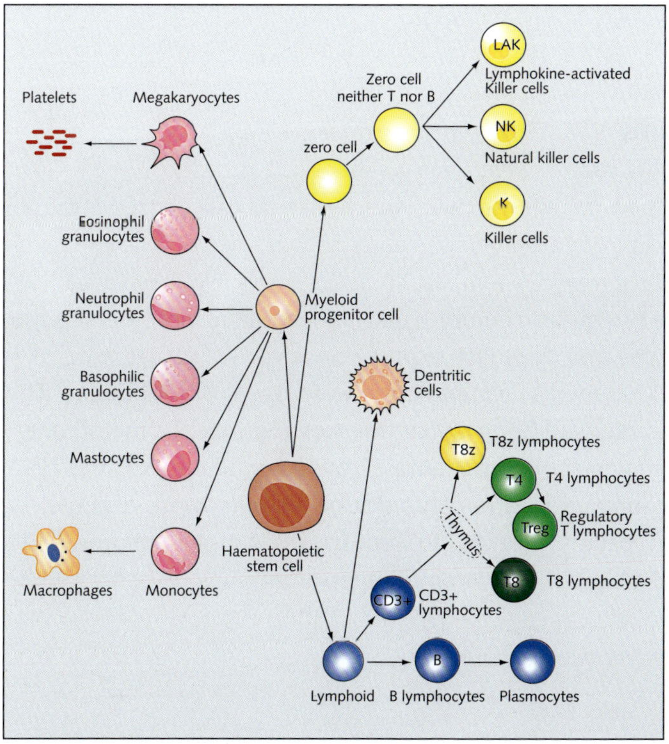

Fig. 1:
Origin of the Immune Cells

Among T lymphocytes, the initial development involves naïve CD3+ lymphocytes, also known as "T3 lymphocytes." They are referred to as "naïve" because they have not yet undergone thymus-mediated maturation. The effector functions of T lymphocytes originate from these naïve cells and are divided into CD4+ and CD8+ lymphocytes, known as T4 and T8 lymphocytes, respectively. B lymphocytes are also produced in the bone marrow. The name "B lymphocytes" originated from their discovery in birds, where they are produced by a gland in the intestine called the bursa fabricii. Plasma cells or plasmacytes, which develop from B lymphocytes, are the effector B lymphocytes responsible for the humoral immune response. They produce specific antibodies targeted against viral or bacterial antigens, contributing to antigen-specific immune defense.

Apart from T and B lymphocytes, natural killer cells or NK cells develop from the hematopoietic stem cell via the null cell. These cells represent a distinct subgroup of lymphocytes that defend against pathogens in a nonspecific manner.

The dendritic cell holds a unique role in immune cell development. It also originates from the hematopoietic stem cell and is commonly referred to as an "antigen-presenting cell." Collaborating with T and B lymphocytes, the dendritic cell facilitates antigen-specific immune defense.

4.2 Defence Mechanisms

As previously mentioned, the immune defense mechanisms can be categorized into two distinct types:

Non-specific or innate immune response: The non-specific immune response is the first line of defense against pathogens and does not require prior exposure or learning. It is a rapid and generalized response aimed at eliminating a wide range of pathogens. The innate immune system includes physical barriers like the skin and mucous membranes, as well as various cellular and molecular components. These components, such as neutrophils, macrophages, natural killer cells, and complement proteins, work together to identify and eliminate foreign invaders. The innate immune response is not specific to pathogens but provides immediate protection until the specific immune response can be activated.

Specific or acquired immune response: The specific immune response, also known as the acquired immune response or adaptive immune response, is a highly specialized defense mechanism that develops after exposure to specific pathogens or antigens. Unlike the innate immune response, the specific immune response is characterized by specificity, memory, and the ability to distinguish between self and non-self. This response involves lymphocytes, particularly B and T lymphocytes. B lymphocytes produce antibodies that can recognize and neutralize specific antigens, while T lymphocytes coordinate cell-mediated immune responses and directly eliminate infected or abnormal cells. The acquired immune response has the remarkable ability to "remember" encountered pathogens, enabling a quicker and more efficient response upon subsequent exposures.

By functioning in tandem, the non-specific and specific immune responses provide a comprehensive defense against a wide range of pathogens, contributing to the overall immune system's effectiveness.

4.3 Non-Specific Immune Defence

The non-specific immune response is activated in infections caused by bacteria and can be divided into cellular and humoral defense (from Latin [h]umor = moisture, also juice, liquid). The humoral immune system, which relies on plasma proteins rather than cells, plays a significant role in this response. The humoral immune system consists of specific and non-specific components. The non-specific defense is primarily mediated by the complement system, while the specific defense involves immunoglobulins (such as IgA and IgG).

The cellular defense is executed by natural killer cells (NK cells), macrophages, and neutrophil granulocytes, which are types of phagocytes (cells that engulf and destroy pathogens). When a germ enters the skin through a wound, macrophages quickly intercept it. These macrophages release various cytokines, including IL-1, IL-2, and TNF-a, which help recruit more macrophages. This cellular response also involves the release of cell adhesion molecules, allowing eosinophilic and neutrophilic granulocytes to enter the capillaries and reach the site of the wound. Macrophages and neutrophil granulocytes work together to destroy the protein coat of bacteria and eliminate them.

Bacteria that remain outside of cells are eliminated locally through the cellular response (as shown in the left side part of Figure 2).

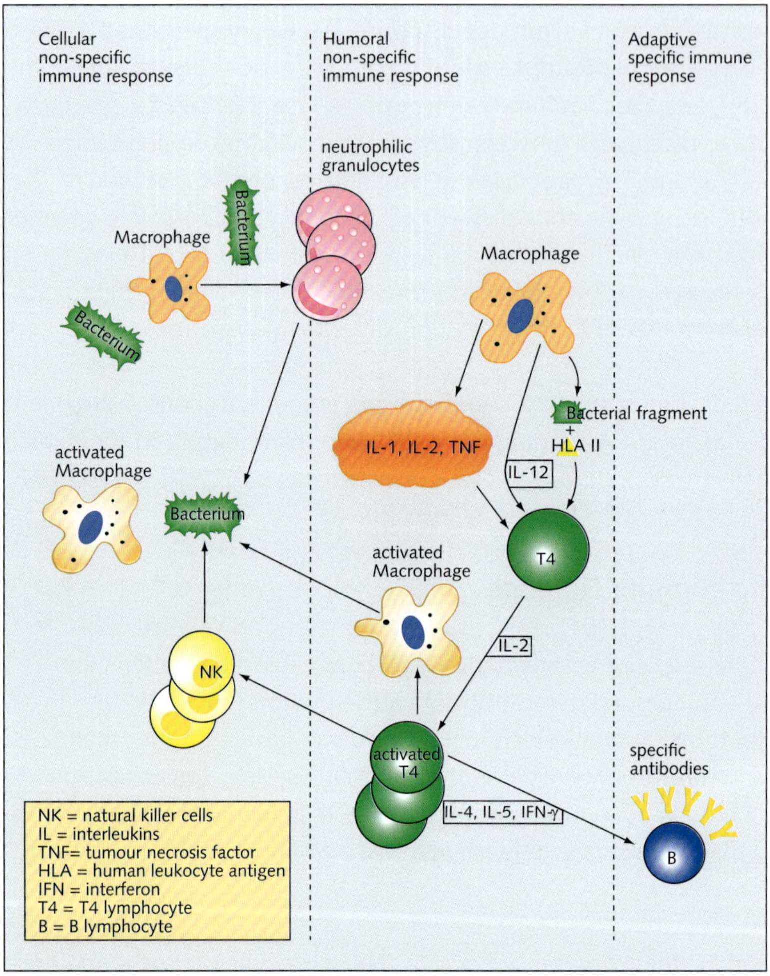

Fig. 2:
Non-Specific Immune Defence

The immune system operates as a complex network with fluid transitions between its components. If bacteria invade cells (intracellular infection) or in cases of reinfection, another immune response is activated known as the humoral (adaptive) response. Macrophages present a bacterial antigen (a piece of protein) together with a molecule called HLA[17] class II to T4 lymphocytes. These T lymphocytes, in turn, activate other T lymphocytes through the release of interleukin-2 (IL-2), as well as additional macrophages that exhibit stronger activity against the bacteria (as depicted in the lower part of the diagram).

17 The term "HLA" (Human Leukocyte Antigen) is explained on page 95.

An activated T cell differs from other T lymphocytes in that it has encountered an antigen, while the others remain inactive.

Extracellular pathogens include streptococci, staphylococci, Neisseria, Escherichia coli, Klebsiella, fungi, and parasites. In these cases, only bacterial proteins can be detected in the blood, and specific antibodies against the bacteria, such as streptolysin[18] in streptococci, are not yet present.

In the case of intracellular bacterial pathogens like Borrelia, Chlamydia, Rickettsia, etc. (as seen on page 19), macrophages act as antigen-presenting cells, and an adaptive immune response, which involves the production of specific antibodies, occurs. These antibodies are produced in a subsequent step by activated B lymphocytes (as shown in the middle and right side part of ▶ Figure 2).

Following an immune response, macrophages clean up any remaining protein envelopes, leaving the site of the event without further traces.

4.4 Specific or learned Defence

During a e.g., viral infection or reinfection, a learned or adaptive immune response is initiated, involving different mechanisms compared to bacterial infections.

Viruses are obligate intracellular parasites that require host cells to replicate. Infected cells become pathogenic, meaning they are diseased cells. The humoral defense, which involves the production of antibodies, primarily works against viruses that are outside of cells. However, once viruses have entered host cells and established an intracellular infection, the cytotoxic T8 lymphocytes play a crucial role. These T8 lymphocytes are responsible for identifying and eliminating virus-infected cells, even if it means damaging the body's own cells. This process is known as cytolysis, and it can be considered an autoimmune or auto aggressive immunological response since it involves the destruction of the body's own cells.

18 Streptolysin is a protein in the cell walls of Streptococcus pyogenes with haemolytic activity. It is released during inflammatory infections by streptococci and is an exotoxin that dissolves (lyses) red blood cells. After an infection, antibodies form against streptolysin O, which are called "antistreptolysin O".

In the adaptive immune response to viral infections, several key steps occur:

1. Recognition of infected cells: The immune system must identify cells that have been infected by a virus. Infected cells often display viral antigens on their surfaces, which can be recognized by specific immune cells.
2. Activation of cytotoxic T lymphocytes (T8 cells): Upon recognition of infected cells, cytotoxic T8 lymphocytes are activated. These T8 cells have the ability to directly kill virus-infected cells.
3. Destruction of infected cells: Activated T8 lymphocytes release cytotoxic molecules, such as perforin and granzymes, which induce apoptosis (cellular self-destruction) in the infected cells. This process helps limit viral replication and spread.
4. Memory response: Following the clearance of the infection, a population of memory T cells is generated. These memory T cells "remember" the specific viral antigens and mount a more rapid and effective immune response upon re-exposure to the same virus in the future.

While the immune response to viral infections can lead to the destruction of infected cells, it is a crucial defense mechanism to prevent the spread of the virus. The immune system's ability to distinguish between healthy and infected cells helps minimize damage to the body's own tissues.

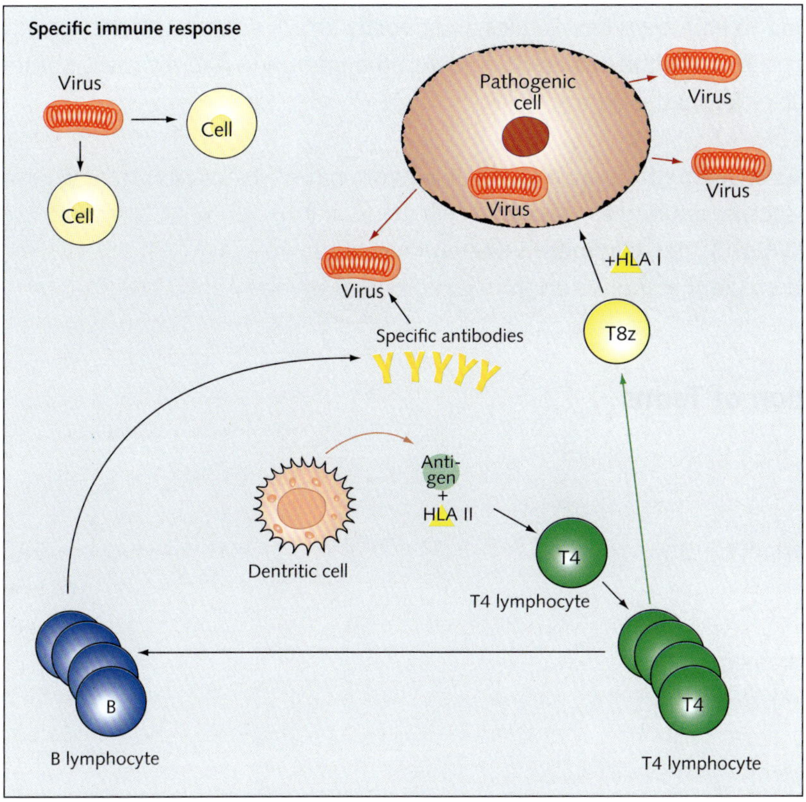

Fig. 3: Specific Immune Defence

In the Specific or learned defence, B lymphocytes play a crucial role by producing specific antibodies that target the viral antigens. Once the viral invader is successfully fought off, the specific immune response is terminated. However, memory cells persist in the immune system, enabling a rapid activation of new B lymphocytes and the production of specific antibodies in case of a subsequent viral infection or reactivation.

In the specific immune defense, dendritic cells take on the task of antigen presentation. They present viral antigens to T4 lymphocytes using HLA class II molecules. This interaction triggers the activation of additional T4 lymphocytes and B lymphocytes, which produce specific antibodies. Simultaneously, T8 lymphocytes are activated. These T8 lymphocytes, along with HLA class I molecules, directly target and destroy virus-infected cells through their cytotoxic activity.

During a primary infection or vaccination, the cytotoxic T8 lymphocytes are particularly important. They bind to HLA class I molecules and directly attack antigens or pathogenic cells. These cytotoxic T8 lymphocytes are considered the immune system's most potent weapon for Specific or learned defence.

Overall, the specific or learned defence involves a coordinated response where B lymphocytes produce specific antibodies, dendritic cells present antigens to T4 lymphocytes, and cytotoxic T8 lymphocytes eliminate infected cells. The presence of memory cells ensures a swift and efficient response upon re-exposure to the same viral antigen.

4.5 Explanation of Terms

Cellular Defence

Innate immune response in the sense of "cells eat bacteria".

Humoral Defence

It can be innate and learned. Certain immune cells secrete messenger substances such as cytokines. Since these proteins are present in soluble form, one also speaks of "humoral", i.e., "concerning the bodily fluids".

Adaptive Defence

In the case of a bacterial infection, specific antibodies are also produced by the B lymphocytes for a short time. The immune system is flexible and reacts briefly to e.g., intracellular pathogens. However, no learned immunity develops afterwards.

Specific or learned defence

An antibody response that originates from memory cells when there is a new intracellular or viral infection or viral reactivation.

5 Immune System Network

The immune system operates as a self-contained network that responds to both external and internal stimuli. It reacts to various factors, including pathogens, hormones, and psychological influences. It is crucial to recognize that within this control loop, altering a single component will inevitably lead to changes in all other elements of the system as well.

5.1 A Short Introduction to the Use of a Network

Many years before I wrote a guide with ten rules[19] for the IT department of a major bank on network management, later I realized that the same principles can be applied to the immune system. The immune system, like a network, is interconnected within the cellular, organ, and overall human system, which in turn is connected to the broader environment, the world, and the universe.

Drawing inspiration from the IT field, the author I recognized the value of looking at things from a different perspective. The concept of multitasking, where multiple processes or programs run simultaneously, mirrors the constant activity of our human body. Every day, every minute, and even every second, our body engages in numerous tasks simultaneously.

Similarly, in a network, programs run concurrently and interact with one another. Information is exchanged between programs, processed, and then the programs continue their execution. This parallel and interconnected nature is also observed within our immune system, where various components work together to defend against pathogens and maintain overall health.

19 "Brevier für vernetztes Denken" © Corinne I. Heitz for UBS-ORKI, May 1991 (slightly modified to explain the system "human being").

The Whole and the Parts

To comprehend a system, it is necessary to recognize its individual components without dismantling them. The focus should be on understanding the interaction among these components, rather than solely observing their isolated actions. For the system to effectively and securely fulfil its purpose, all parts must harmoniously integrate and work together.

Interconnectedness

Wholeness arises from the interaction among individual parts within a system. This interaction can take various forms, including circular relationships that are not strictly based on cause-and-effect, but rather on circular patterns. These relationships are depicted in a network, where correlations exist in both the same and opposite directions. Negative feedback loops contribute to stability, while positive feedback loops can either amplify or lead to collapse.

One potential pitfall when analysing networks is the tendency to isolate individual parts and their relationships without fully acknowledging their impact within the larger whole. This approach fails to recognize the significant influence of the parts within the network and their interconnectedness with one another.

The System and its Environment

The categorization of what constitutes a part, a system, or an environment depends on the perspective of the observer and the chosen frame of reference. Systems, by their nature, are open and interconnected with their surrounding environment. They exist as components within a larger system, forming a hierarchical structure of nested systems. Each system within this hierarchy can be viewed as a part from one perspective and as a whole from another, depending on the chosen frame of reference. Thus, the classification of entities as parts, systems, or environments is context-dependent and subject to the observer's viewpoint.[20]

20 It has been shown that the environment has a greater influence on the immune system than the genetic make-up. Source: Petter B., Vladimir J. et al.: Variation in the Human Immune System Is Largely Driven by Non-Heritable Influences. http://www.cell.com/cell/abstract/S0092-8674%2814%2901590-6 [retrieved 16.3.2021].

Complexity

The distinction between complexity and complication is important. A complex system is characterized by its dynamic nature, in contrast to a static system. It exhibits a wide range of behaviours and interactions among its components. Analytical methods often fail to provide accurate predictions for complex systems, as their behaviour is highly non-linear and influenced by numerous factors. Instead, empirical values and observations are essential for understanding and controlling complex systems. By studying the system's behaviour through practical experience and real-world data, effective control strategies can be developed. It is through this empirical approach that the intricacies of complex systems can be navigated and managed.

Order

While not all elements within a system are connected to every other element, many connections do exist among various components. A system possesses its unique structure, exhibiting a specific pattern of behaviour that distinguishes it from other systems. It is through this order and organization that expectations can be formed regarding the system's behaviour. Understanding and influencing a system necessitates grasping its inherent order and comprehending how its components interact.

By studying the system's structure and the relationships between its elements, one can gain insights into its functioning. This understanding enables us to anticipate and shape the system's behaviour according to our objectives. Recognizing the order within a system is vital for effective analysis, intervention, and control.

Steering

Goal-oriented behaviour involves taking proactive measures to intervene in a system before undesirable consequences arise. It goes beyond a reactive approach of waiting for deviations to occur and then responding. Instead, control over a system is achieved through deliberate steering and pre-emptive actions.

Waiting for deviations to manifest can lead to unexpected outcomes and make it challenging to regain control. By implementing preview and goal-oriented steering, one can anticipate potential deviations and take preventive measures to mitigate or avoid them

Micro-Immunotherapy plays a significant role in this process. It involves using targeted therapies to support the immune system's response against viruses or bacteria associated with autoimmune diseases. By providing the immune system with the necessary tools and support, Micro-Immunotherapy helps the immune system regain control and restore balance.

In this context, Micro-Immunotherapy can be described as an "order therapy." It aims to restore order and harmony within the immune system by facilitating a balanced immune response to the triggers associated with autoimmune diseases.

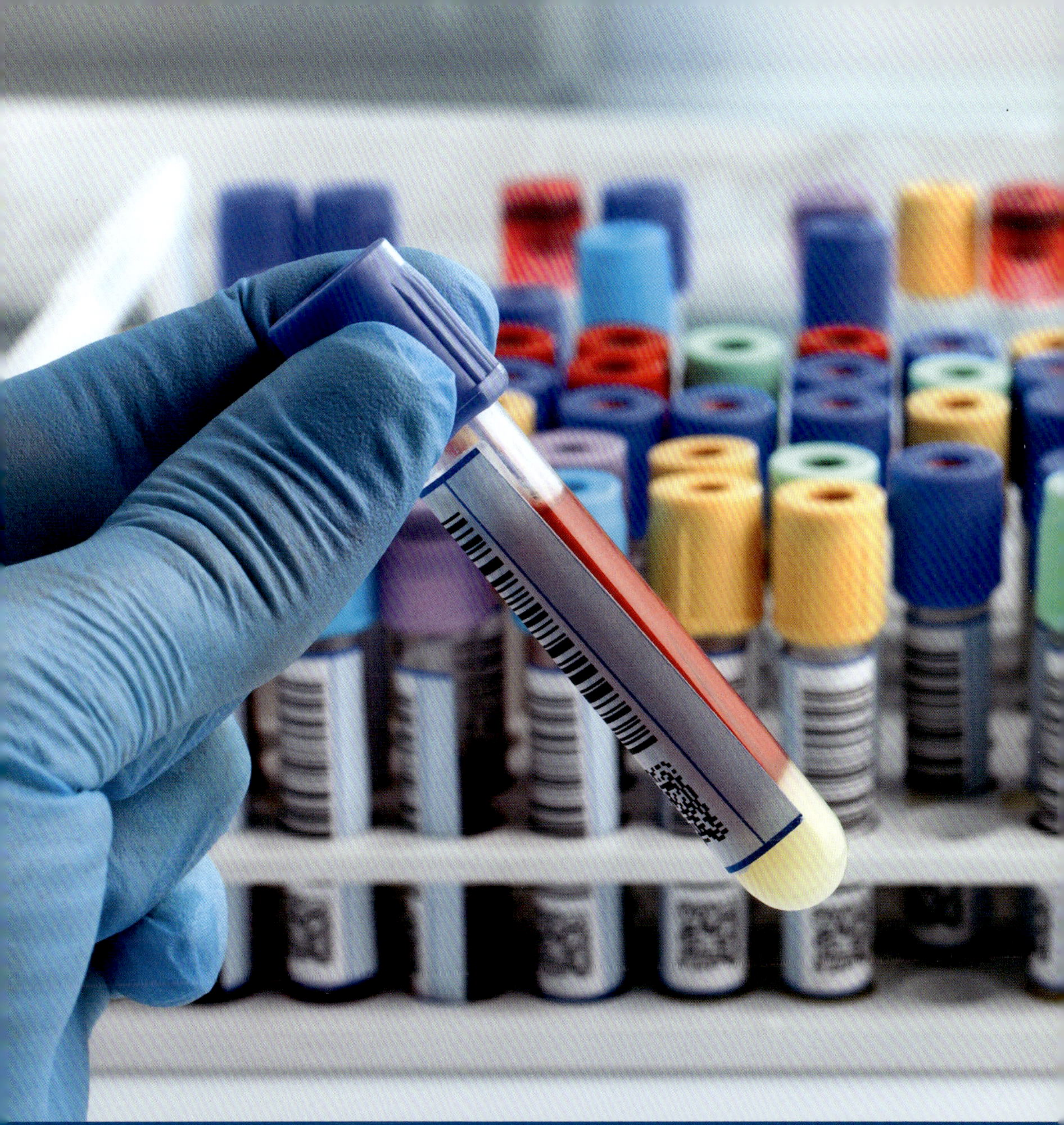

Practical Part

6 Medical History

An accurate analysis of a patient's condition is built upon a thorough anamnesis, which forms the foundation of the diagnostic process. There is no such thing as a "wrong" or "right" anamnesis, but it is crucial not to overlook any pertinent information. It is not uncommon for patients to have extensive medical records filled with various examinations that have not yielded a definitive diagnosis.

In such cases, it suggests that relevant aspects may have been missed during the examinations. Some medical practices provide anamnesis forms for patients to complete before their initial consultation. While this approach aims to gather important information, rigidly predefined forms run the risk of overlooking essential details that may only come to light during a conversation between the patient and the healthcare provider.

Structuring the questioning and examination process can be immensely helpful. Both the therapist and the patient should understand that conducting a comprehensive anamnesis takes time. The procedure recommended by the author in their practice has been effective, but it is essential for each healthcare provider to develop their own approach in engaging with patients and obtaining the necessary information.

It is important to emphasize that open and attentive communication, as well as active listening, are crucial during the anamnesis. By taking the time to gather a comprehensive history, healthcare providers can ensure that no significant details are overlooked, leading to a more accurate analysis and subsequent treatment plan.

6.1 Conversation

First, let the patient tell the story calmly:

- all symptoms (physical and psychological)
- first occurrence,
- Weight and size
- Operations
- previous diseases
- Diseases in the family
- Vaccinations
- Accidents
- social status (e.g., married, in partnership, living alone)
- Leisure activities, sports etc.
- unfulfilled desire to have children
- Number of children
- Occupation and job satisfaction.

Specific questioning by the therapist to identify symptoms that indicate possible diseases:

1. *What Happened Shortly (3-6 months) Before the First Appearance of the Main Symptoms?*
    - z. e.g., flu-like infection
    - Accident
    - Divorce
    - Loss of a loved one
    - Stress in the family or at work.

2. *Skin*
    - Temperature, cold, warm
    - dry, wet
    - Sweating, freezing
    - Skin colour, e.g., yellowish, tanned pale, scaly
    - Redness
    - Pustules
    - Rashes
    - Acne
    - cold sores
    - Hair
    - Finger and toenails.

3. *Digestion*
    - Diarrhoea
    - Constipation
    - Frequency of bowel movements
    - Cramps
    - Tenesmus
    - Reflux, heartburn
    - Stomach, intestinal pain
    - Haemorrhoids.

4. *Joints and Muscles*
    - Pain
    - when?
    - with or without load?
    - Swelling
    - Mobility.

5. *Cardiovascular*
    - Angina pectoris
    - Varicose veins
    - Palpitations, heart palpitations
    - Blood pressure.

6. *Neurological Complaints*
    - Motoric skills
    - fine motoric skills
    - Neuralgia
    - Paraesthesia
    - Tingling
    - restless legs
    - Paralysis.

7. Sensory Organs

- Eyes
- Sense of smell
- Sense of taste
- Hearing.

8. Sleeping Habits

- enough sleep
- awake in the morning or
- long start-up time
- Exhaustion
- Midday nap
- Difficulty falling asleep or staying asleep.
- when they go to bed and how many hours of sleep

9. Performance

- Exhaustion physically or psychologically
- Concentration disorders
- Hyperactivity.

10. Allergies and Intolerances

11. Women Additionally:

- Regularity of menses
- PMS
- Menopause
- Interdiction
- Course of pregnancies and births
- Abortions (spontaneous or intentional).

12. Men Additionally:

- Difficulty urinating
- strength of the urine jet
- Erectile dysfunction
- Interdiction.

6.2 Everyday Behaviour and Further Information

1. Eating Habits

- Mixed diet
- vegan, vegetarian
- organic
- keto
- fastening

2. Drinking Quantities (Water)

3. *Stimulants and Addictive Substances*
   - Coffee
   - Alcohol
   - Nicotine
   - Drugs
   - Energy drinks
   - Stimulants.

4. *Current Medication Intake incl. Natural Remedies, Food Supplements and Homeopathy.*

5. *Dental Status (Recent Panoramic Image)*[28]

6. *Previous Therapies and all Previous Laboratory Results as Well as Findings, X-Rays, MRI Reports, etc.*

7. *Family Situation*

A detailed anamnesis is crucial for formulating precise requirements for laboratory diagnostics. It helps in developing an initial hypothesis that can then be confirmed through laboratory tests and potentially other diagnostic procedures.

This process requires considerable experience and intuition. Healthcare providers need to engage with patients directly, physically examining them by touching the skin, palpating for pain, and assessing tissue changes. Basic knowledge of manual techniques is also beneficial for identifying malposition, postures, and working with structures such as tendons, muscles, and joints.

In the case of chronic and autoimmune diseases, it is common to test for Herpesviridae, which are reactive viruses. These tests help determine if the presence of these viruses is contributing to the patient's condition.

By combining the information obtained through a thorough anamnesis with appropriate laboratory and other diagnostic tests, healthcare providers can develop a comprehensive understanding of the patient's condition and tailor treatment plans accordingly.

It is important to note that laboratory testing and diagnostic approaches may vary depending on the specific case and the suspected underlying causes.

28 If a patient presents with an occlusion disorder (malocclusion), the focus may not necessarily be on searching for pathogens responsible for back pain. Instead, it could be beneficial to establish a strong therapeutic network to refer the patient to a holistic dentist.

7 Laboratory Diagnostics

7.1 Designated Laboratories

In the context of Micro-Immunotherapy, the Adaptive Defence is not solely on determining the viral load, but rather on identifying viral reactivation. Therefore, it is crucial to obtain accurate and therapeutically relevant laboratory results.

In regions like ours, it is common to find the presence of herpes viruses in a large proportion of the population. Simply receiving a result stating the presence of herpes virus type 1 or 2 without further context or specific details is not particularly useful.

For Micro-Immunotherapy, specific laboratory values are required to guide treatment effectively. These values are further explained in detail within the text. Medical associations[29] have collaborated to identify and evaluate specialized laboratories with the necessary quality standards. This ensures consistent standards for all healthcare providers. The addresses of these approved laboratories can be found in the appendix for reference. (Refer to page 181).

29 Medical association for Micro-Immunotherapy for German speaking countries: https://MeGeMIT - Medizinische Gesellschaft für Mikroimmuntherapie MeGeMIT.org
INternational: https://www.micro-immunotherapy.com/

8 Serology

The term "serology" encompasses all tests that can be performed on a patient's blood serum. In the context of Micro-Immunotherapy, certain parameters are particularly relevant and commonly analysed.

As standard serological tests for Micro-Immunotherapy, the following antibodies are commonly performed:

- EBV
- HHV-1: Herpes simplex virus type 1 (HSV-1) and 2
- Varicella Zoster
- Cytomegalovirus
- Toxoplasma gondii

8.1 Epstein-Barr Virus

Among the viruses of the herpes family, the Epstein-Barr Virus (EBV) holds particular relevance in chronic diseases. Understanding its significance requires a brief digression.

HHV-4: Epstein-Barr Virus (EBV) is a common virus that infects a large portion of the population worldwide. It is primarily transmitted through saliva, and most people are exposed to EBV at some point in their lives. In most cases, the infection causes mild symptoms or goes unnoticed. However, in some individuals, EBV can lead to more severe health issues and long-term consequences.

EBV has been linked to various chronic conditions, including infectious mononucleosis (commonly known as "mono" or glandular fever), as well as certain types of cancer, such as Burkitt's lymphoma, Hodgkin's lymphoma, and nasopharyngeal carcinoma. Moreover, emerging research suggests potential associations between EBV and other autoimmune and neurological disorders, such as multiple sclerosis and chronic fatigue syndrome.

The relevance of EBV in chronic diseases is underscored by the substantial number of scientific articles available on the internet discussing the importance of EBV[30]. This abundance of literature indicates the significant research interest and ongoing investigations into understanding the role of EBV in various health conditions.

30 Retrieved 7.3.2021 A search revealed approximately 820,000 scientific articles on EBV.

In the context of Micro-Immunotherapy, addressing EBV and its potential implications may be a crucial aspect of treatment. Testing for EBV-specific markers and assessing the immune response to the virus can help guide therapeutic interventions and personalized treatment plans.

HHV-4: Epstein-Barr Virus (EBV) has probably been with mankind since its inception.

Studies exploring the genetic variations of the Epstein-Barr Virus (EBV) in different ethnic groups have provided insights into how the virus interacts with the human immune system and its potential impact on health outcomes. These studies have shed light on the complex relationship between EBV, genetics, and disease manifestations.

It has been observed that certain genetic variations in individuals can influence their immune response to EBV infection. This includes variations in genes related to human leukocyte antigen (HLA)[31] , which plays a crucial role in the immune system's recognition and response to foreign substances. Different HLA (p. 95) alleles have been associated with varying susceptibilities to EBV-related diseases.

As therapists we are challenged and must always expect that our patients inform themselves on the internet. Within our work, it is important not to overestimate EBV. It has been proven that EBV promotes certain types of cancer, such as Hodgkin's and non-Hodgkin's lymphomas, Burkitt's lymphomas and certain types of leukaemia. Reactivation of EBV does not automatically imply that a person is terminally ill or destined to develop a severe condition. Many individuals experience EBV reactivation without significant health consequences.

The global research efforts focused on developing vaccines against Epstein-Barr Virus (EBV) have brought increasing attention to the potential risks associated with the virus. Institutions such as the renowned Helmholtz Centre[32] have also directed their research towards understanding the implications of EBV.

"EBV is an extremely successful virus; almost 98 percent of all adults are infected with it. Most infections occur in childhood predominantly without symptoms. The first infection in adolescents or adults, on the other hand, leads in about 50 per cent of all cases to

31 Rajiv Khanna, Robert W. Slade, Leith Poulsen, Denis J. Moss, Scott R. Burrows, John Nicholls and Jaqueline M. Burrows: Evolutionary dynamics of genetic variation in Epstein-Barr virus: Isolates of diverse geographical origins: Evidence for immune pressure independent genetic drift. Journal of Virology, 1997 Nov; 71(11): 8340-8346

32 Helmholtz Zentrum München German Research Center for Environmental Health (GmbH)

mononucleosis, which usually heals completely in healthy people, but can sometimes take a severe course or become chronic.

EBV was also identified as the first human tumour virus. It is responsible for the development of about 200,000 cases of cancer worldwide every year. The virus is particularly dangerous for people with a weakened immune system, such as AIDS patients or transplant recipients. They often contract EBV-caused lymph node cancer and post-transplant lymphoproliferative disorders (PTLD), which often lead to death. For this risk group in particular, vaccination before transplantation could drastically reduce the risk of PTLD.[33]"

It is important to differentiate between the reactivation of Epstein-Barr Virus (EBV) and a chronically unhealed primary infection. Reactivation of HHV-4: Epstein-Barr Virus (EBV) tends to occur when the body is weakened or becomes Adaptive Defence, such as during periods of trauma, serious accidents, or high levels of stress (both psychological and physical). Consequently, it is not uncommon for high-performance athletes to experience EBV reactivation, which can lead to a significant decline in their performance.

Recent research has revealed that EBV has the ability to interact with the human genome. EBV persists within our DNA and potentially induce epigenetic changes. This suggests that EBV has the capacity to influence gene expression and cellular function in ways that may contribute to the development or progression of certain diseases.

Laboratory Diagnostics for EBV

The following values are required:

- EBV VCA (Virus Capside Antigen) IgG
- EBV VCA IgM
- EBV EBNA (EB nucleid antigen) IgG
- EBV EA (Early Antigen) IgG

Indirect immunofluorescence (IF) remains the preferred method for analyzing reactivations in Micro-Immunotherapy, as it provides the necessary linear readings to accurately identify reactivations, not only for Epstein-Barr virus (EBV)[34]. In comparison to the detection method of ELISA (enzyme-linked immunosorbent assay), IF offers distinct

33 http://www.helmholtz-muenchen.de/jahresbericht2011/forschungshighlights/13_f_2_5.html [retrieved 13.6.2015] Original in German, translated by the Author

34 Despite multiple tests, there have been no new results available for the other laboratory kits aimed at achieving precise determination. It was initially anticipated, even during the first edition's publication, that the indirect immunofluorescence method would be replaced by more advanced and precise methods in the near future.

advantages that make it indispensable in Micro-Immunotherapy. IF enables a linear interpretation of the values, which is not achievable with ELISA.

▶ *The Following Simple Rules Apply to the Interpretation of the EBV:*

The immune response to EBV takes place in three steps.

First, antibodies of the IgM class are formed. If IgM is positive, we talk about an acute first infection, also called "Mononucleosis". Later, antibodies against the virus capsid antigen (protein coat of the virus) of the IgG class are added.

The so-called "early antigens" are directed against the infected cell. They arise before the replication of the DNA, which is why they are called "early" antigens. They always indicate reactivation. The detection of HHV-4: Epstein-Barr Virus (EBV) early antigens (EA) is associated with increased morbidity. For instance, in a study involving 26 adults and 18 children below the age of 15 who presented with a range of persistent illnesses and symptoms, such as chronic neck pain, fever, headache, lymphatic swelling, depression, myalgia, and fatigue syndrome, the presence of EBV early antigens was observed.[35]

Subsequently, antibodies are generated against other components of the virus, specifically the EBV nuclear antigens (EBNA) known as EBNA-1 to 6. These antigens are only produced following the destruction of B lymphocytes that have been infected with EBV. The presence of EBNA antibodies can be equated with the immunological conclusion of a primary infection with EBV.

If EBV VCA IgG and EBV EA IgG as well as EBV EBNA IgG are positive:
▶ There is a reactivation of EBV.

If EBV VCA IgG is positive and EBNA IgG negative:
▶ There is a primary infection with EBV that has not yet been completed.

While EBV VCA IgG indicates the primary infection, EBNA stands for a passed and completed EBV infection.

35 Jones JF, Ray CG, Minnich LL, Hicks MJ, Kibler R, Lucas: Evidence for active Epstein-Barr virus infection in patients with persistent, unexplained illnesses: elevated anti-early antigen antibodies, Ann Intern Med. 1985 Jan;102(1):1-7.X DO Source: http://www.ncbi.nlm.nih.gov/pubmed/79029 [accessed 9 Mar 2021].

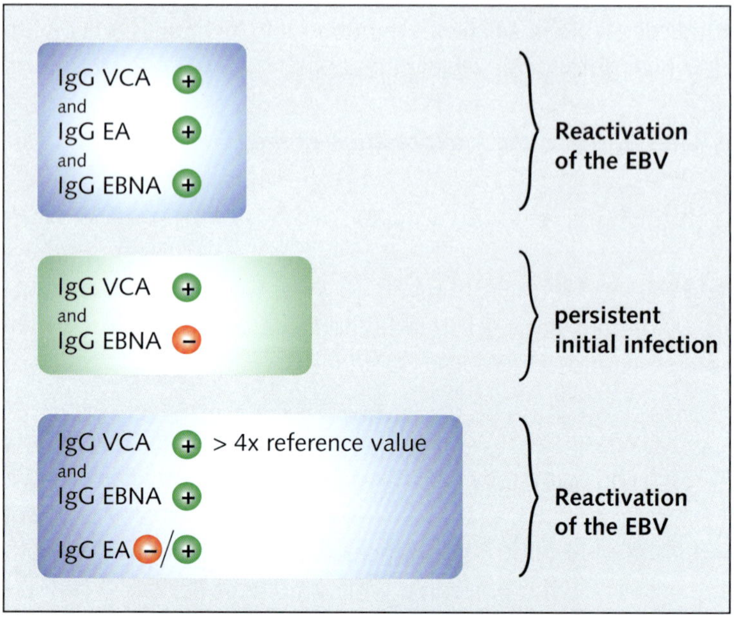

Fig. 4: EBV Serology

As long as EBNA IgG is negative, the infection persists. If EBNA is missing, we talk about a chronic persisting mononucleosis. EBNA can also be lost secondarily - this indicates an incompetent or deficient immune system (e.g., under immunosuppression).

Even when both HHV-4: Epstein-Barr Virus (EBV) VCA IgG and EBV EBNA IgG tests yield positive results, it can still be classified as a reactivation, but only if the titer is at least four times higher than the reference value.

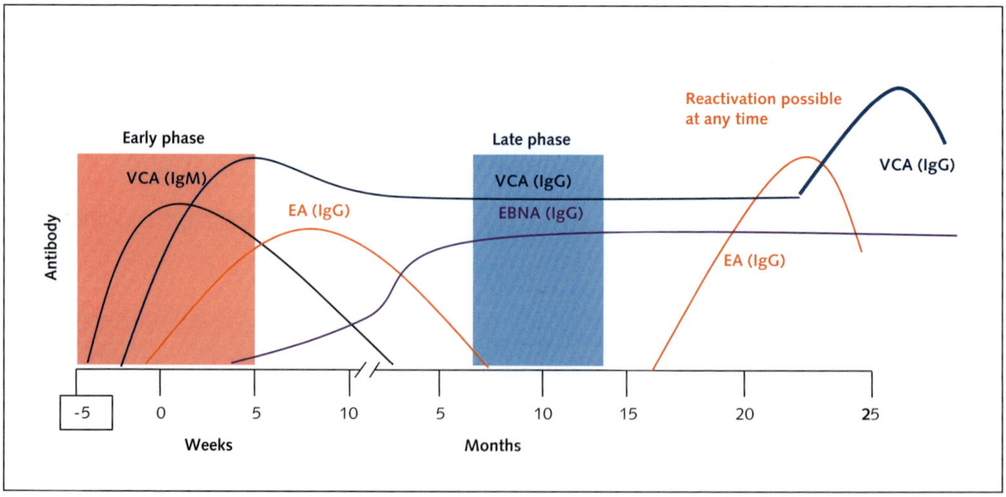

Fig. 5: Course of the Disease EBV (Mononucleosis)

To accurately determine the extent of virus titer increase, it is crucial to compare the obtained results with the reference value provided by the respective laboratory. This reference value serves as a baseline for assessing the magnitude of the virus titer elevation.

If the reference value for HHV-4: Epstein-Barr Virus (EBV) VCA IgG is, for example, 80, then:
1 : 160 2 times
1 : 320 3 times
1 : 640 4 times
1 : 1280 5 times

8.2 Herpesviridae

- HHV-1: Herpes simplex type 1 (HSV-1) and
- HHV-2: Herpes simplex type 2 (HSV-2)
- HHV-3: Varicella-zoster virus (VZV)
- HHV-5: Cytomegalovirus (CMV)
- HHV-6: Human Herpes Virus 6,
- HHV-7: Human Herpes Virus 7 and
- HHV-8: Human Herpes Virus 8
- IgG quantitative or IF
- IgM
- IgA

Interpretation

1. IgG Positive or Elevated in ELISA:

Shows a previous infection, reactivation is possible if there is a quantitative measurement available, and the obtained value is significantly higher than the specified index or reference value. This indicates a substantial increase in viral activity and suggests the occurrence of a reactivation.

2. IgG Elevated in IF:

If the value is at least 4 times higher than the reference value, reactivation can be assumed.

3. IgM Positive or Elevated in ELISA and IF[36]

Shows a fresh infection.

36 Depending on the laboratory, results are obtained from ELISA or indirect immunofluorescence.

8.3 Toxoplasma Gondii

Toxoplasmas are obligate intracellular protozoa. In order to make any definitive statement about the infection, a quantitative determination is necessary. Without quantitative data, it is challenging to provide meaningful information regarding the extent or severity of the infection.

Toxoplasma IgG-AB	IgM -AB	Interpretation
low	low	persistent infection
high	low	subsiding infection
high	high	recent infection
low	high	acute infection

Other Pathogens

Further examinations are initiated based on the patient's symptoms (see pathogens p. 12).

8.4 Bacteria

In case of a bacterial infection, the presence of IgG indicates either a current or past infection. Generally, bacterial infections (extracellular) do not leave immunological traces in the form of antibodies (IgG), leading to the absence of immunity. However, there is an exception with intracellular bacteria (refer to page 16). IgG levels can remain elevated for an extended duration without causing pathogenic effects, although the specific titer level plays a certain role.

Example

Chlamydia serology

Chlam. trach. IgA-AB (IFT)	negative	<1:40
Chlam. trach. IgG-AB (IFT) ↑	**1:80**	<1:80

While one might assume that a positive IgG result indicates a past infection, it is important to note that a recent infection cannot be completely ruled out. Therefore, the laboratory includes the following explanation:

"Serologically, the presence of IgG suggests either a remote past infection or an early stage of an acute infection. If the clinical presentation aligns with this possibility, it is advisable to follow up with another examination in approximately two weeks or consider pathogen detection through PCR" (PCR refer to footnote on page 120).

To obtain definitive proof, it is necessary to perform a swab test, such as a urogenital or ocular swab. These swabs can provide conclusive evidence in confirming the infection.

Chlam. pneum. IgA-AB (IFT)	**1:320**	<1:80
Chlam. pneum. IgG-AB (IFT)	**1:640**	<1:80
Chlam. pneum. IgM-AB (IFT)	**↑1:10**	<1:10

In contrast to the previous example, this result is significant. With IgM positive (negative would be <10) we find a primary infection. Since IgG and IgA are also strongly elevated, a persistent infection can be assumed.

Treatment is always mandatory in the presence of elevated IgA and/or IgM values. If only IgG is elevated, all other serology values must also be taken into consideration.

9 Interpretation of Immune Status

The term "immune status" refers to a lymphocyte typing specifically designed for Micro-Immunotherapy. Special attention was given to presenting the various values in a graph format to facilitate interpretation. It should be noted that the graphs may differ among reference laboratories (refer to appendix on page 181). While internal laboratory structures are challenging to modify, laboratories must adhere to scientific guidelines. The graphs utilized in this context are those provided by Viollier AG laboratory in Basel Switzerland, because it combines almost all values in one Graph. The diagram was developed in collaboration with the author, drawing on years of practical experience, input from the International Association for Micro-Immunotherapy, and the expertise of various laboratories.

This immune status is also available from Lab4more if you specify "Immune status Switzerland" in the request. Since more parameters than usual are requested, this costs somewhat more at Lab4more.

At LADR Baden-Baden, the immune status "2IDI" or "new" can be requested. The activated T-lymphocytes are then subdivided into T3 act, T4 act and T8 act, while the NK-lymphocytes are summarised in one bar.

Depending on the question, it may be interesting to get a different evaluation. For oncological topics it is more important to see the subgroups of natural killer lymphocytes, for general questions the activated T-lymphocytes can be interesting.

The immune system consists of leukocytes and lymphocytes and the subpopulations of the latter. These are T3, T4, T8 as well as B lymphocytes and natural killer cells. In addition, there are regulatory T-lymphocytes and some essential subclasses (see ▶ Figure 6).

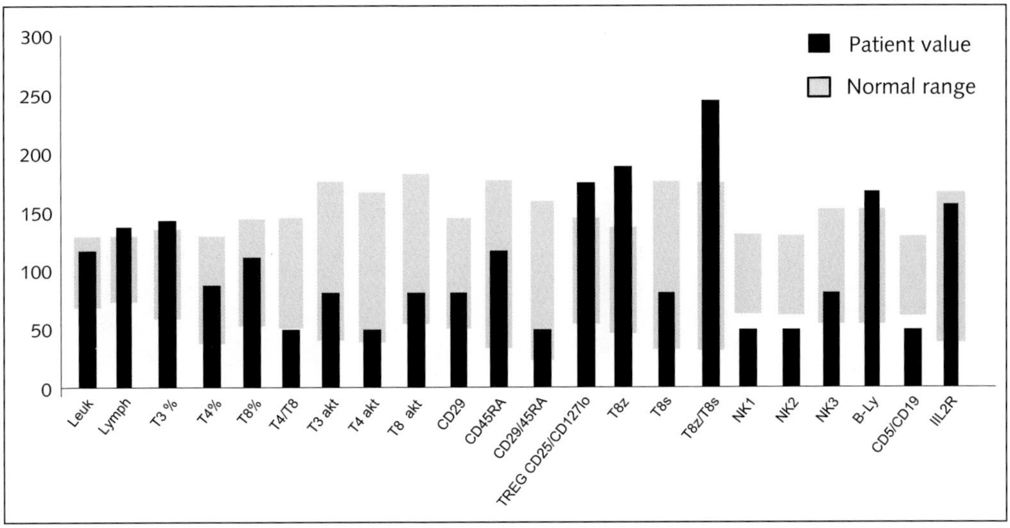

Fig. 6: Lymphocyte Typing

The graph can be used to draw certain immunological and therapeutically relevant conclusions, which is why the order of the values in the graph is important.

The graph shows the "should be" values with a grey background, the black bars correspond to the patient values.

9.1 Leukocytes

A first aspect we look at is the total number of leucocytes and lymphocytes.

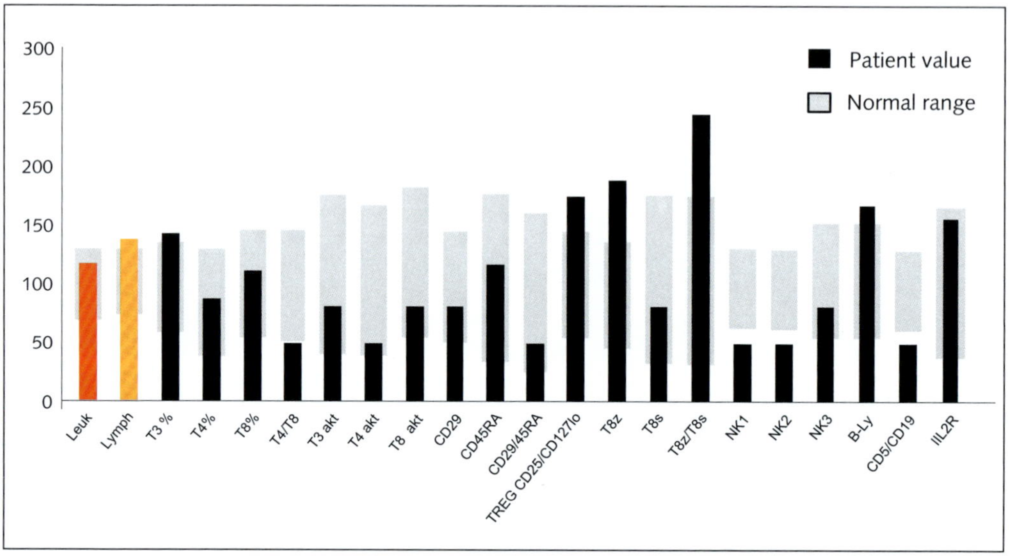

Fig. 7: Leukocytes / Lymphocytes

The leucocytes are also divided into various subgroups, one of which is the lymphocytes. It is useful to look at these first.[37] The leucocytes are divided into:

Designation	Reference Value
Leukocytes	G/L 4.5 – 11.5
Neutrophil granulocytes	G/L 1.40 – 8.00
Eosinophil granulocytes	G/L <0.70
Basophilic granulocytes	G/L <0.20
Monocytes	G/L 0.16 – 0.95
Lymphocytes	G/L 1.50 – 4.00

37 Any hemogram, commonly utilized in most doctors' cabinet, can provide these values within a matter of minutes.

Elevated leukocyte levels are often associated with infection or inflammation, although this assumption is not always accurate. Changes in leukocyte count do not necessarily provide insights into the state of the immune system. Nevertheless, they do offer valuable clues regarding the appropriate direction for further diagnostic investigations:

- Allergy,
- Infection,
- Neoplasia,
- Parasites,
- EBV infection.

9.1.1 Granulocytes

Neutrophil Granulocytes

An elevation in neutrophil granulocytes can indicate an infection, inflammation, or neoplasia. Conversely, low levels of neutrophil granulocytes may suggest a potential case of agranulocytosis[38]. Neutrophil granulocytes can be further categorized into:

- segmental granulocytes and
- rod-nucleated granulocytes.

If the segment-nucleated granulocytes are elevated, we talk about a so-called "left shift" in a bacterial infection.

If the rod-nucleated granulocytes are elevated, one speaks of a "right shift", as occurs, for example, with iron deficiency.

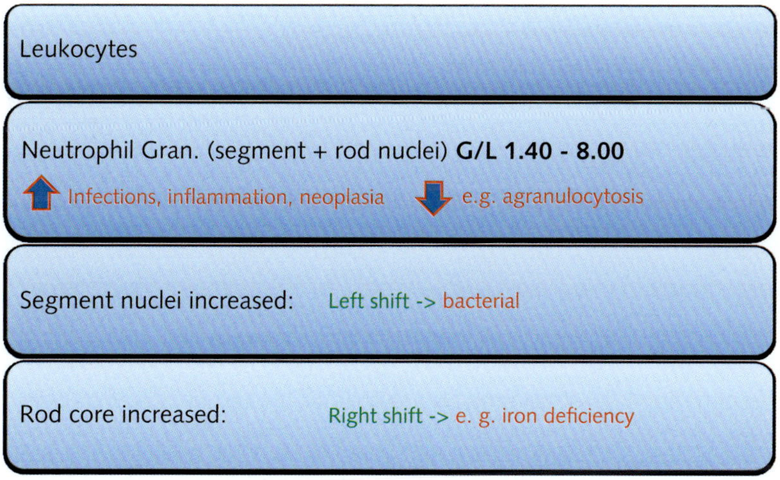

Fig. 8: Neutrophil Granulocytes

38 A severe reduction of granulocytes is usually caused by toxins; drugs and radioactive radiation are possible causes.

Eosinophil Granulocytes

are increased with:	are lowered at:
• Allergies and • Parasites (worms, ticks, fleas) • Fungi	• the acute phase of an infection • Cushing's syndrome • Stress

Basophilic Granulocytes

are increased with:	are lowered at:
• Allergies • Parasites (worms, ticks, fleas) • Fungi • endocrine metabolic diseases • Hyperlipidaemia	• Elevated cortisol levels and • Stress

9.1.2 Monocytes

are increased with:	are decreased with:
• Monocytosis, classic in EBV infection • chronic infections • Autoimmune diseases	• e.g., aplastic anemia

9.2 Lymphocytes and Subpopulations

9.2.1 Aspects of Interpretation

Different names for different lymphocytes often make understanding difficult. The author only uses the term "lymphocytes" instead of "cells" for the following purposes: e.g., T4-lymphocytes and not the term "cells", such as T4-cells. The term "CD" means "cluster of differentiation" and is used for human antigens. Thus, T3 lymphocytes have a positive cluster of differentiation 3 and are thus also called "CD3+ lymphocytes or cells".

The lymphocytes, along with their subgroups, are integral components of leukocytes and collectively constitute what we refer to as the "immune system."

In the initial stage of interpretation, it is essential to ascertain whether the immune system is hyperreactive or hyporeactive, indicating an over- or under function, respectively. This aspect plays a crucial role in determining the appropriate therapy.

The total count of lymphocytes is assessed, representing the overall number of lymphocytes involved in immune defence. If this count is abnormally low, it indicates a condition of general or primary immune hypo reactivity. This state is characterized by lymphopenia, which refers to a deficiency or lack of lymphocytes.

If the total lymphocytes are elevated, we speak of a hyperactive immune system.

Before we go into details, let's first get an overview. The number of lymphocytes is decisive, without knowledge of the significance of the individual subgroups.

1. Aspect of Interpretation

If the total lymphocyte count exceeds the normal range, it indicates a state of general or primary immune hyperreactivity. This condition is characterized by lymphocytosis, which refers to an excessive number of lymphocytes.

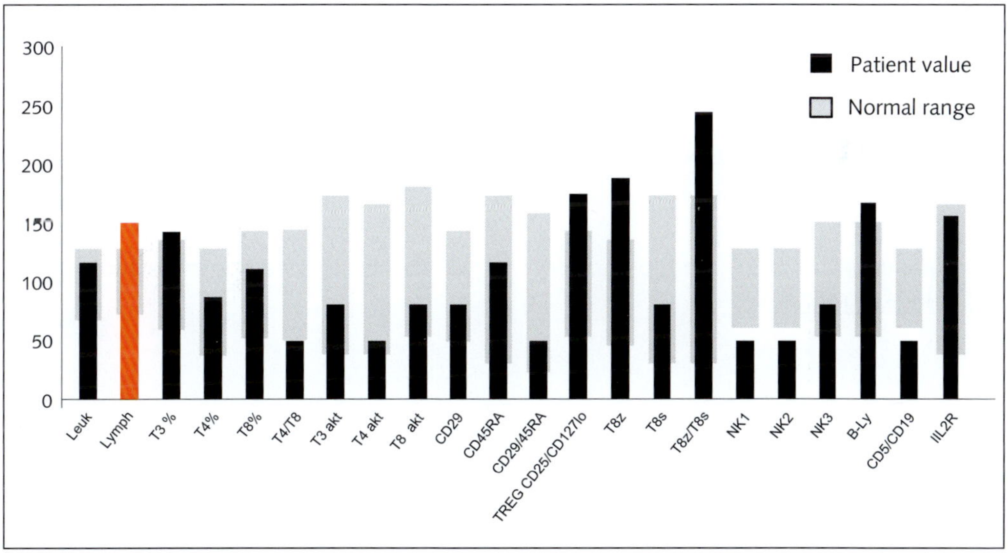

Fig. 9: Total Lymphocytes

In children, an increase in lymphocytes is considered the norm until puberty.

2. Aspect of Interpretation

FIf neither lymphopenia nor lymphocytosis is present, we will look at the main categories (T3, T4, T8) of immune cells and their activation. The following graph shows that although the T3 lymphocytes are increased in percentage, the activated T3, T4 and T8 lymphocytes are below normal. This immune system is therefore hyporeactive.

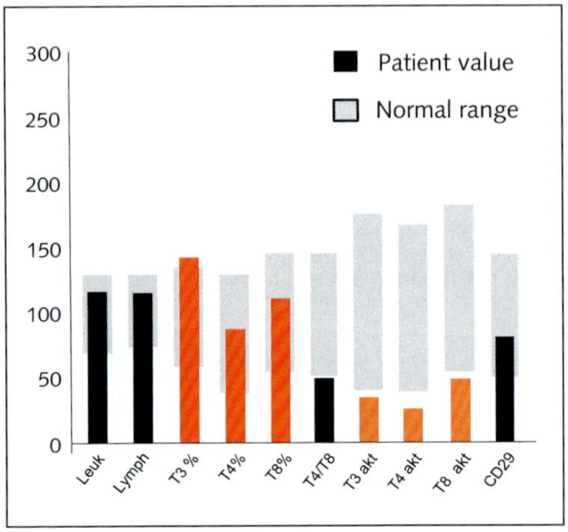

Fig. 10: Hyporeactive Immune system

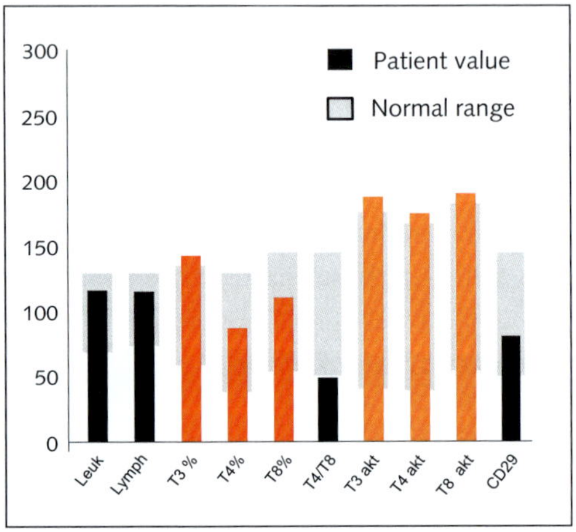

Fig. 11: Hyper-reactive Immune system

If the levels of activated T-lymphocytes exceed the normal range, it indicates a hyperreactive immune system. This remains true even if the percentages of T3, T4, and T8 lymphocytes are within or below the normal range, as long as the total lymphocyte count falls within the normal range.[39]

The distinction between a hypo- or hyperreactive immune system is important for the right choice of therapy.

39 This interpretation deviates from the previous understanding that reduced levels of T3, T4, or T8 cells indicate hyporeactivity, while increased levels indicate hyperreactivity. It has been acknowledged that the decisive factor is the presence of activated T-lymphocytes. This approach is particularly relevant in the context of autoimmune events since only activated T-lymphocytes possess immunocompetence.

9.2.2 When is the Immune System HYPER- or HYPO-active?

An immune system with reduced lymphocytes is HYPO-active
An immune system with increased lymphocytes is HYPER- active If the lymphocytes are in the norm, a distinction is made between:

- Adaptive = the activated T lymphocytes are in the norm
- Reactive = the activated T lymphocytes are above the norm
- Secondary hypo-reactivity = activated T-lymphocytes are below the norm

Additional Rule of Thumb:

1. If one of the following parameters is reduced, the immune system is HYPO-active
   - Lymphocytes (total) or decreased lymphocytes
   - Activated T lymphocytes
   - T3 lymphocytes
   - T4 lymphocytes
   - T8 lymphocytes
   - T8z lymphocytes
   - B lymphocytes

2. If **NONE** of the above parameters are decreased, then the following rule applies:
   - If one or more of the above mentioned values is elevated, then the im- mune system is considered as HYPER-active.

The following example illustrates an immune system post-treatment with cytostatics (chemotherapy). In patients with significant immunosuppression or undergoing chemotherapy, performing a lymphocyte typing does not yield meaningful results. This is because chemotherapy destroys a substantial portion of leukocytes, leading to a highly hyporeactive immune system. Due to the sluggish nature of the immune system's recovery process, it takes approximately six months for certain characteristics to become detectable through lymphocyte typing. Therefore, it is advisable to wait until this period has elapsed before conducting the typing. However, this waiting period does not apply before initiating therapy for an impaired immune system.

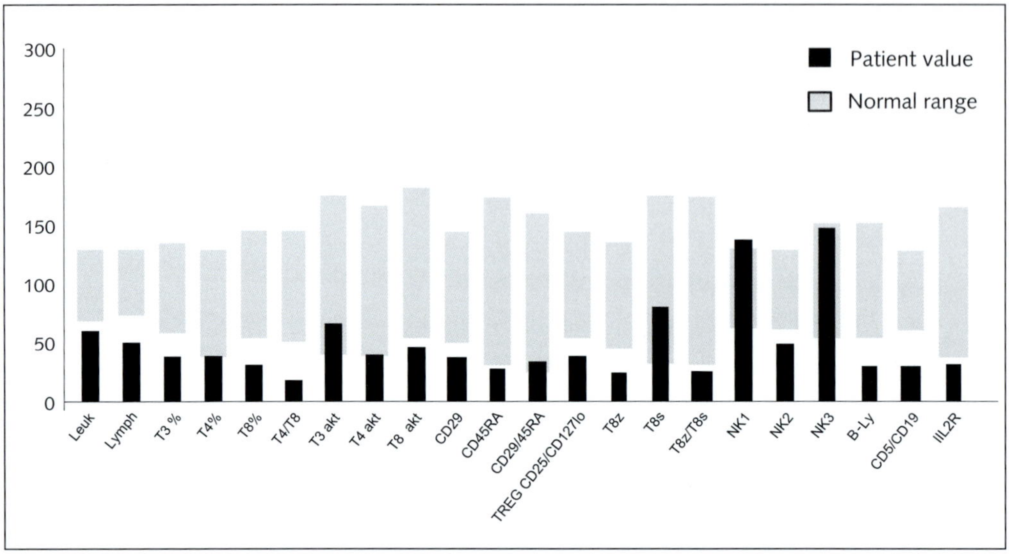

Fig. 12 Deficient Immune System

9.3 Importance of Lymphocytes

Once the initial determination of hyperreactive or hyporeactive immune system has been made, the significance of lymphocyte subgroups comes into play.

9.3.1 T3 Lymphocytes

T3 lymphocytes are immature (naive), not yet differentiated cells. They will become B, T4 or T8 lymphocytes.

An increase in T3 lymphocytes is found with an increased need for T4, T8 cells and B lymphocytes. A decrease in T3 lymphocytes should not be observed, as it would indicate an inactive immune system.

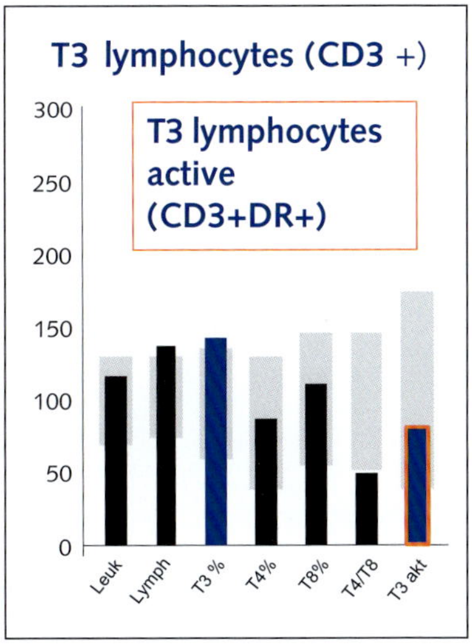

Fig. 13: T3 and activ T3 Lymphocytes

▶ *Activated T3 Lymphocytes*

During the late/follow-up phase, T3 lymphocytes become activated and express HLA-II receptors (HLA = Human Leucocyte Antigens) for antigen presentation.

CD3+DR+ positive lymphocytes serve as an indicator of the current activity level of the immune system. A decreased lymphocyte count is indicative of a reduced active immune system.

When viral or bacterial processes are present, a decrease in both T3 lymphocytes and activated T3 lymphocytes indicates a failure of the immune response.

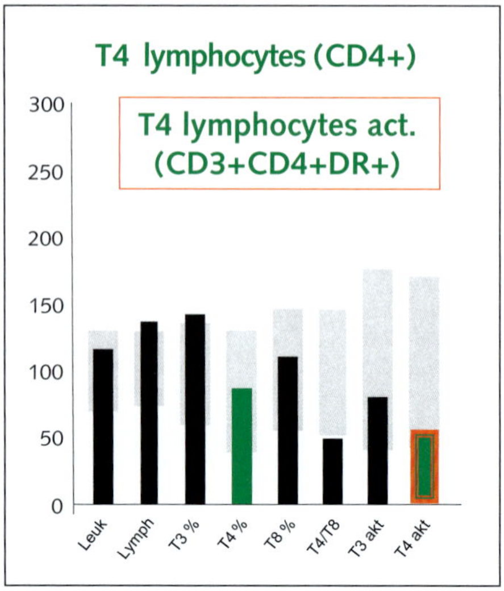

Fig. 14: T4 and activ T4 Lymphocytes

9.3.2 T4 Lymphocytes

T4 lymphocytes rest in the lymph nodes and are ready for activation.

T4act are activated T4 lymphocytes they have come into contact with the antigen presenting cell and an antigen and a class II HLA molecule.

An elevated count of activated T4 lymphocytes is indicative of a viral event. Conversely, a high number of naive[40] T4 lymphocytes with a low proportion of activated T4 lymphocytes suggests an extracellular infection, such as a bacterial infection, or an allergic reaction.

High proportions of activated T3 and T4 lymphocytes are found, for example, in non-responders after vaccinations which indicates a high activity of the immune system.

40 Non-activated T-lymphocytes are also called "naive".

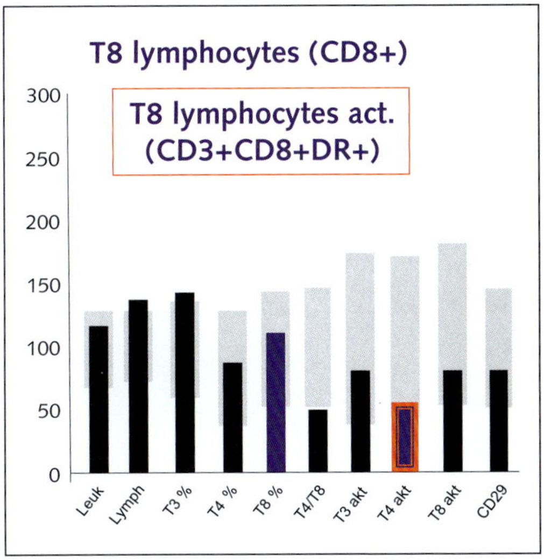

Fig. 15: T8 and activ T8 Lymphocytes

9.3.3 T8 Lymphocytes

T8 lymphocytes that have not yet been activated and rest in the lymphoid organs.

A decrease in T8 lymphocytes (refer to page 84) accompanied by an increase in T4 lymphocytes suggests a bacterial infection, parasites, or an allergic condition.

Activated T8 lymphocytes have contacted antigen-presenting cells and an antigen as well as a class I HLA molecule. All endogenous cells produce class I HLA.

A heightened proportion of activated T8 lymphocytes indicates significant immune activity in this context.

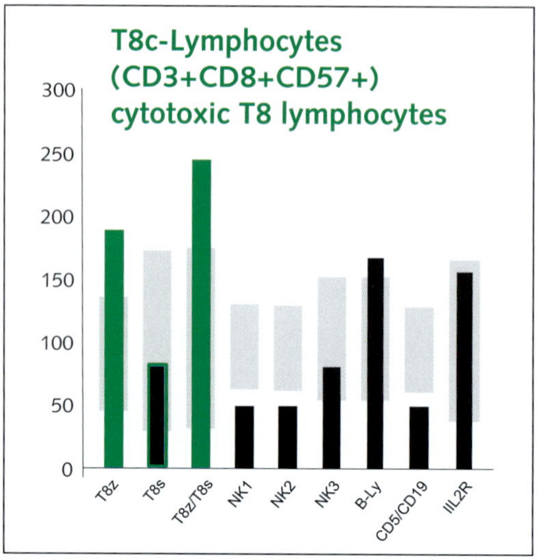

Fig. 16: Cytotoxix T8 Lymphocytes

9.3.4 T8c Lymphocytes (CD3+CD8+CD57+)

The presence of pathogenic cells, such as cancer cells, or intracellular pathogens, especially viruses, leads to an increase in cytotoxic T8 lymphocytes.

A low level of T8c lymphocytes with a simultaneous viral load, such as Epstein-Barr Virus (EBV), indicates a deficiency in immunocompetence.

9.3.5 Killer Cells

Killer cells are particularly important for diagnostics as well as for the therapy of cancer. In cancer patients, the total number of killer cells increases significantly.

They arise (refer to ▶ Figure 1, on page 25) from the Zero cell and are initially neither T nor B lymphocytes.

A further distinction is then made:

1. Natural Killer Cells (NK)

The NK cell is a lymphocyte capable of directly dissolving specific pathogenic cells without requiring prior activation.

NK cells target virus-infected cells and cancer cells. Their cytotoxic activity is regulated by two types of surface receptors: activating receptors and inhibitory receptors. These receptors interact with HLA class I molecules present on the surface of the target cells.

The precise mechanism of target cell recognition is not fully understood. However, it is known that an NK cell binds to a surface glycoprotein on the target cell through its own glycoprotein. The recognition of HLA class I molecules on the target cell provides a signal that inhibits the destruction of the target cell by the NK cell.

However, cells that possess the target cell structure recognized by NK cells but have downregulated HLA-I complex are susceptible to destruction. This phenomenon occurs in certain tumor cells or virus-infected cells. The downregulation of HLA-I complex reduces the inhibitory signal to NK cells, allowing them to carry out their cytotoxic activity against these cells.

IL-2 and interferons enhance the activity of NK cells (but do not activate them!). A further distinction is made between three classes of NK cells:

NK1 Cells (CD57+)

Reduced levels of NK1 cells (CD57) serve as an indicator of the degree of immune suppression in chronic infections. Particularly in Borrelia infections, evaluating NK1 cells can be used as a prognostic laboratory parameter.

NK2 Cells (CD56+CD6+)

NK2 cells make up about 10 % of the NK cells. They are mainly found in lymphatic tissue and produce these cytokines very quickly:

- IFNγ
- TNFα
- GM-CSF
- RANTES

NK3 Cells (CD56+CD16+)

NK3 cells constitute approximately 90% of NK cells and exhibit the highest cytotoxic activity. Their numbers notably increase during viral infections, especially in cases of HIV infection where T4 lymphocytes are frequently diminished. However, in chronic hepatitis C infections, the population of NK3 cells may be reduced.

2. Lymphokinin-Activated Killer Cells (LAC)

Lymphokine-activated killer (LAK) cells are phagocytes that possess HLA-independent cytotoxic activity against tumor cells.

9.3.6 B Lymphocytes

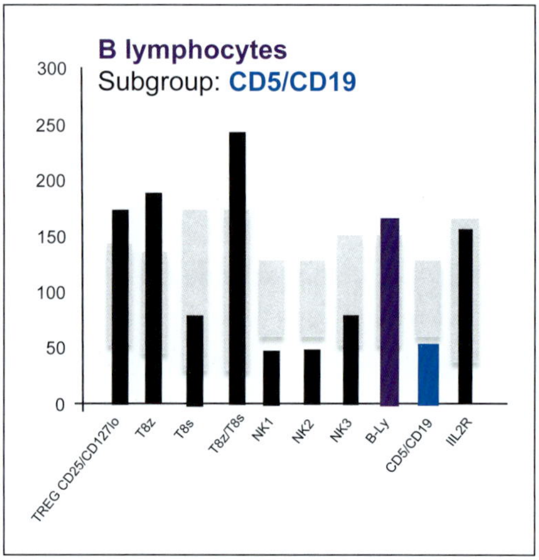

Fig. 17: B Lymphocytes

B lymphocytes, are uniquely capable of producing specific antibodies. They become activated in response to alien antigens and can differentiate into either antibody-producing plasma cells or memory cells. The term "B lymphocytes" was originally coined based on their development in the bursa fabricii in birds. However, in humans and certain other mammals, B cells originate in the bone marrow.

B lymphocytes are initially "antigen-naive", they circulate in the blood and are in the lymph organs.

The process of activation in B lymphocytes begins when the appropriate antigen binds to the B cell receptor. Once bound, the antigen is internalized by the B lymphocyte, broken down, and presented in conjunction with HLA class II molecules on the cell surface as a complex. This complex is recognized by T lymphocytes, which subsequently produce cytokines that ultimately activate the B lymphocytes.

Following activation, B lymphocytes migrate to the germinal centers located in lymph nodes or spleen. Within these germinal centers, the B lymphocytes undergo intense proliferation (division) within the lymph follicles. During this process, the gene segments involved in directing subsequent antibody production undergo rapid cell division. This enables the rapid selection of the most optimal antibody against the invading antigen.

B lymphocytes that have reached their fully differentiated stage and secrete antibodies are referred to as "plasmocytes." These plasmocytes not only secrete specific antibodies but also produce IgE antibodies, as indicated in the serum protein profile on page 88.

A small fraction of activated B lymphocytes undergoes differentiation into memory B cells. These memory B cells effectively "store" the antigen information, enabling a faster and more efficient immune response upon subsequent encounters with the same antigen. This memory response contributes to the enhanced ability of the immune system to mount a rapid and Specific or learned defence during future exposures to the antigen.

An increase in B lymphocytes is observed in:

- B-cell lymphomas, especially chronic lymphocytic leukaemia (CLL)
- Multiple sclerosis
- Graves' disease
- Middle-aged female smokers (often double-nucleated B lymphocytes)
- Progressive sclerosis,
- Stress lymphocytosis (after injuries cardiac emergencies or similar
- Rheumatoid arthritis (untreated, also CD19/CD5-positive subgroup increased)
- Men with anti-sperm antibodies in the serum
- RSV bronchitis in children (also the CD5+ and CD10+ subgroups)

A decrease in B lymphocytes is observed in:

- Heat stroke
- after splenectomy in the past (not confirmed by all studies)
- after intensive training (only relative normalises after 1h)
- after intravenous immunoglobulin G therapy
- after the menopause (as opposed to premenopause)
- in alcoholic cirrhosis of the liver
- with liver carcinoma
- with thymoma
- with iron deficiency

B lymphocytes Subgroup: CD5/CD19
They are a subclass of B lymphocytes, which, when elevated, indicate a tendency toward autoimmune diseases.

9.3.7 Marker

Certain lymphocytes serve as markers for specific immune system developments, provide prognostic information, and indicate the chronicity or activity of a disease.

▸ *Marker CD29*

The CD29 marker plays a role in cell adhesion mechanisms. It is expressed on both CD4+ (T4 lymphocytes) and CD8+ (T8 lymphocytes) T lymphocytes in peripheral blood.

As an activation marker, CD29 indicates a long-lasting activation of the T lymphocytes and is also called "very-late-activation" antigen.

An elevated CD29 marker is indicative of prolonged activation, suggesting a slow and chronic process.

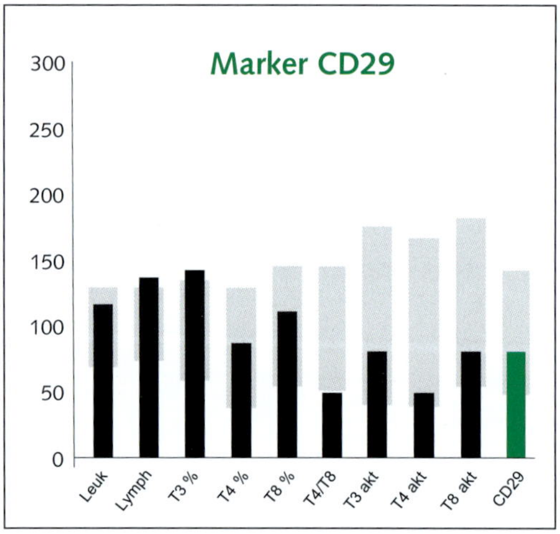

Fig. 18: Marker CD29

▶ *Marker CD45RA*

The CD45RA antigen is found in approximately 50% of (CD4+) T4 lymphocytes (CD4+) and in approximately 75% of T8 lymphocytes, as well as on almost all B lymphocytes and natural killer (NK) lymphocytes. Selective loss of CD4+CD45RA+ has been observed in active multiple sclerosis (loss of antigen on T4 lymphocytes).[41]

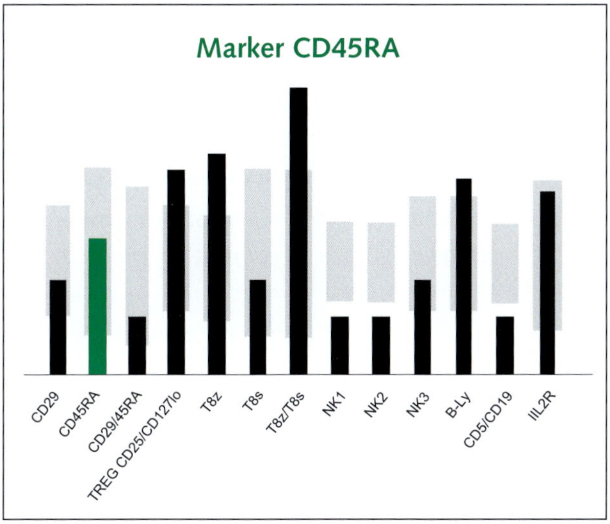

Fig. 19: Marker CD45RA

9.3.8 T-Regulatory Lymphocytes (CD4+-CD25+-T-reg)

Regulatory T lymphocytes (T-reg) play a crucial role in maintaining immune tolerance. They refer to the immune system's ability to distinguish between foreign substances and self-organisms. The immune system combats foreign organisms, while preserving tolerance towards the body's own tissues. The recognition of foreign elements or elements present during the embryonic state is retained as lifelong information.

Immune tolerance should rest in equilibrium. When regulatory T lymphocytes (T-reg) are within the normal range, it indicates normal immune tolerance. However, an increase in the value of T-reg indicates a higher level of immune tolerance, signifying a greater

41 Rose LM, Ginsburg AH, Rothstein TL, Ledbetter JA, Clark EA.: Selective loss of a subset of T helper cells in active multiple sclerosis. Proc Natl Acad Sci USA. 1985; 82:7389-7393.
Sobel R., Hafler D., Castro E., Morimoto C., Weiner H. The 2H4 (CD45R) antigen is selectively decreased in multiple sclerosis lesions. J Immunol. 1988; 140:2210-2214.

capacity of the immune system to prevent self-destruction. While elevated regulatory T lymphocytes (T-reg) can indicate a higher level of immune tolerance, it can also be a sign of cancer cells present in the body. Cancer cells can exploit immune regulatory mechanisms, including T-reg cells, to evade immune detection and avoid destruction by the immune system. In such cases, the immune system may tolerate the presence of cancer cells instead of mounting an effective immune response against them. Monitoring T-reg levels alongside other diagnostic markers can help in assessing the immune response to cancer and evaluating its progression.

On the other hand, a decrease in regulatory T lymphocytes (T-reg) is indicative of an autoimmune event. This is due, in part, to the loss of immune tolerance.

Regulatory T lymphocytes produce interleukin 10 (IL-10), which exerts an anti-inflammatory effect by inhibiting excessive immune system reactions. IL-10 plays a crucial role in controlling and resolving inflammatory responses as well as promoting the development of immune tolerance.

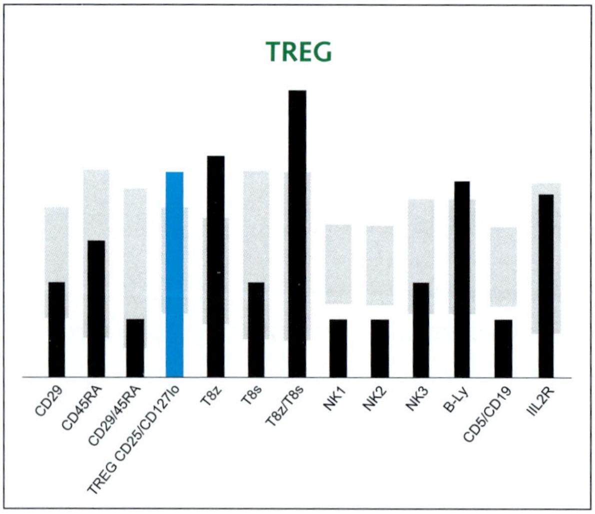

Fig. 20: Regulatory T Lymphocytes

9.3.9 Soluble IL-2 receptor in serum

It is widely recognized that T lymphocytes play a central role in the immune system. One of their primary functions is to uphold cellular immunity, particularly in response to intracellular persistent pathogens such as viruses, some bacteria, and cancer cells.

Interleukin-2 (IL-2) is a key cytokine involved in T-lymphocyte activation. It plays a crucial role in stimulating T lymphocytes to undergo division and carry out their functions. However, it is worth noting that quantitatively measuring IL-2 levels in the serum has not demonstrated significant diagnostic relevance.

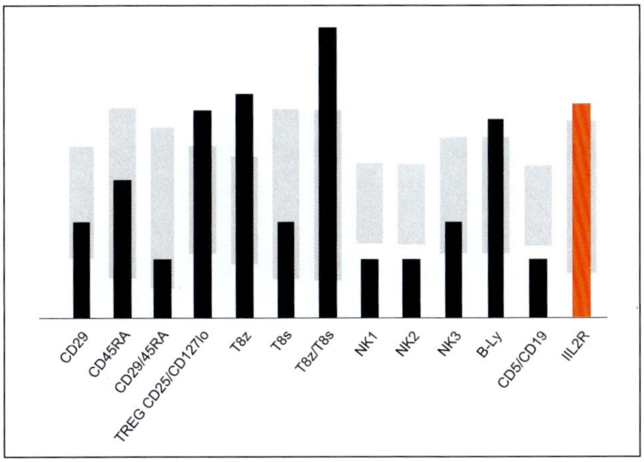

Fig. 21: Interleukin-2 Receptor

"For quantification of lymphocytic activation, the soluble IL-2 receptor is now available. The binding of Interleukin-2 to the IL-2 receptor on the lymphocyte surface provides the actual activation stimulus for the T lymphocyte.

IL-2-activated lymphocytes increase the number of membrane-bound IL-2 receptors and simultaneously release a soluble form (soluble IL-2 receptor = sIL2R) into the blood. The function of sIL2R is to bind excess IL-2 and release it later (depot effect). The sIL2R is measurable at a low level in the serum of healthy individuals and significantly increases in a range of diseases associated with T-cell activation. Unlike global markers of inflammation such as CRP or ESR, the sIL2R specifically and rapidly indicates the activation of the patient's T lymphocytes, making it suitable for the diagnosis and monitoring of these immunologically mediated diseases.

A high sIL-2R thus indicates high immunitary activity and is thus also a marker for autoimmune diseases."[42]

42 Source: http://www.imd-berlin.de/fachinformationen/diagnostikinformationen/loeslicher-IL-2-rezeptor-im-serum.html [retrieved: 16.3.2021] Translation from German to English by the Author

9.3.10 TH-17

T-helper lymphocytes 17 (TH17) produce interleukins IL-17 and IL-22. IL-17 is responsible for autoimmune diseases and acts as an inflammatory factor, playing an important role in antimicrobial defence against fungi. The previously accepted, strict TH1/TH2 model is challenged by TH-17. While TH17 cells are pro-inflammatory similar to IFN-γ-producing TH1 cells, they are more associated with chronic inflammatory processes. Efficient TH1 (IFN-γ) immune responses are suppressed by IL-17, leading to the persistence of the pathogen or antigen and thus the chronicity of the immune reaction (chronic infection, autoimmune diseases).

TH17 cells also express IL-22, which likely plays a role in coordinating both innate and adaptive immune responses. Therefore, maintaining a balance between T-reg and TH-17 cells is crucial.

When immune tolerance is diminished (low T-reg and high TH-17), it can result in severe autoimmune reactions.

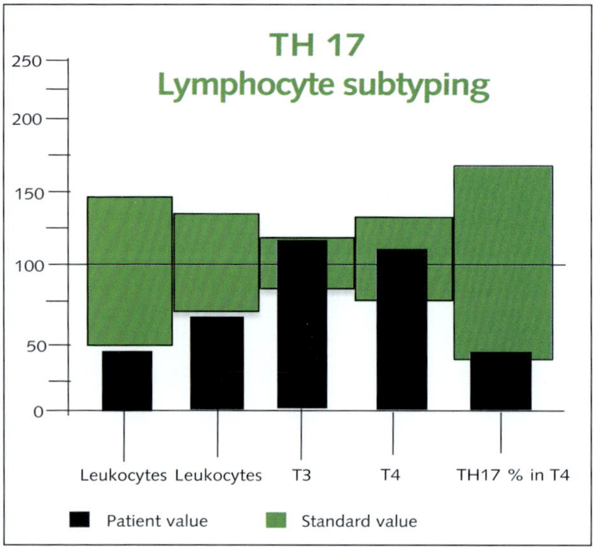

Fig. 22: TH 17

TH-17/T-Reg

It is interesting to consider the balance between TH-17 and T-reg cells. Similar to TH1 and TH2 cells, TH-17 and T-reg cells should be in balance. TH-17 and T-reg cells exhibit antagonistic behavior, meaning:

- Increasing T-reg cells leads to a decrease in TH-17 cells, and vice versa.
- T-reg cells are responsible for immune tolerance and immune self-tolerance.
- Increasing T-reg cells strengthens tolerance and simultaneously reduces TH-17 cells, thus reducing autoimmunity. However, it also increases the risk of a cancerous process.
- Conversely, a decrease in T-reg cells corresponds to reduced tolerance, which is associated with autoimmune processes. If at the same time, TH-17 cells are elevated it is also an indication of autoimmune diseases.

9.3.11 TH1/TH2 Cytokine Status

Cytokines are the messengers of the immune system (refer to page 106). Depending on their distribution and release, they perform various tasks within the immune system. The most important key cytokines are:

the TH1 response:

- IL-2
- IFN-gamma
- TNF-α

and the TH2 response:

- IL-4
- IL-5
- IL-10 determined.

TH1 Response:

These cytokines are involved in the cellular immune response and stimulate the activities of T lymphocytes.

TH2 Response:

These cytokines primarily influence the humoral immune response, which involves the production of specific antibodies and the development and proliferation of B lymphocytes.

TH1/TH2

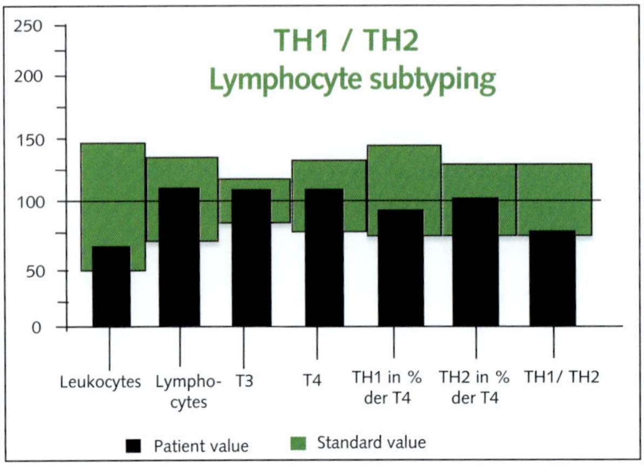

Fig. 23: TH1 / TH2

TH1

DTH1 lymphocytes are a subgroup of T4 lymphocytes. They play a role in regulating inflammatory processes and defense against extracellular pathogens. TH1 lymphocytes interact with antigen-presenting cells and a molecule of the HLA class II.

Macrophages activated by TH1 lymphocytes, through the secretion of interleukin-12, induce the differentiation of T lymphocytes into TH1 lymphocytes.

Interferon-gamma (IFN-γ) is the key effector and cytokine of TH1 lymphocytes. It triggers pro-inflammatory immune reactions. The processes induced by IFN-γ contribute to the efficient elimination of intracellular pathogens (viruses, intracellular bacteria), but in excessive or inadequate responses, they can also cause tissue damage.

TH2

TH2 lymphocytes are also a subgroup of T4 lymphocytes. Their primary function is to execute the class switching of B lymphocytes.

In addition to the primary activation of B lymphocytes, TH2 lymphocytes can induce an isotype switch (class switching of antibodies) in B lymphocytes through the release of specific cytokines.

- IL-4 starts the change from IgM to IgG1 and IgE
- IL-5 starts the change from IgM to IgA

In addition, IL-5 activates eosinophil granulocytes, giving TH2 lymphocytes an important role in the development of allergies and extracellular immune responses, particularly in defence against parasites.

Interleukin-4 (IL-4), like IL-5, is secreted by TH2 lymphocytes. Increased IL-4 synthesis indicates a predominance of the TH2 immune response and is frequently observed in individuals with allergies and certain autoimmune diseases. A TH2 shift also occurs in advanced stages of various chronic infections.

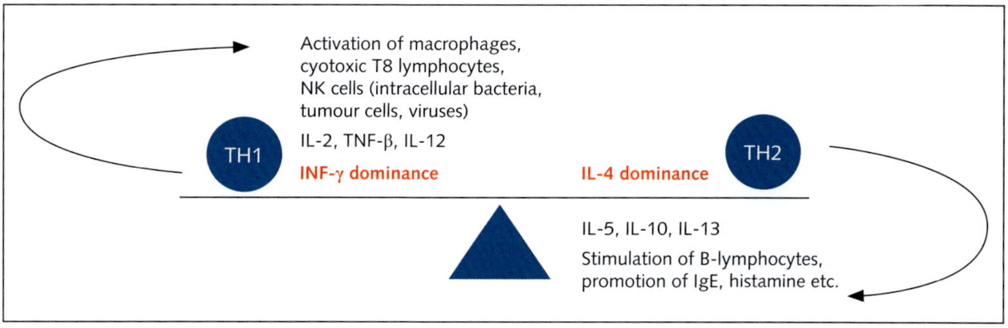

Fig. 24: TH1 / TH2 Balance

TH1/TH2 Ratio

After antigen exposure, T4 lymphocytes are stimulated to proliferate and differentiate into either TH1 or TH2 cells. Depending on their subtype (TH1 or TH2), they produce different cytokines that induce B lymphocytes or plasma cells to produce different classes of immunoglobulins.

TH1 lymphocytes release interferon-gamma (IFN-gamma), which leads to the production of IgG classes 1-3. The TH1 response is involved in defence against bacterial or viral infections.

TH2 lymphocytes produce IL-4 and IL-5. IL-4 stimulates B lymphocytes to produce IgE and IgG class 4. IL-5 activates eosinophil granulocytes and increases IgA production by B lymphocytes. This TH2 response is observed in allergic diseases and parasitic infections.

9.5 Oncological Aspects

In cases of immune incompetence, T8 suppressor cells increase while cytotoxic T8 lymphocytes remain decreased. This corresponds to a poorly regulated viral infection or a pre-cancerous condition (resembling a pyramid, without illustration).

Oncologist Dr. Gerhard Hubmann in Vienna has extensively studied oncological patterns in immune status. He reaches the following conclusion:
"*When T8 lymphocytes and/or T8s lymphocytes are revved up, resembling a plateau or staircase, the system is giving gas with the handbrake on. If this occurs only in one branch of T8 or T8s lymphocytes, it indicates an old pathogen burden. However, if both branches of T8 lymphocytes and T8s lymphocytes increase, they appear as 'vampire fangs' (see Figure 27, page 87), which indicates a deep-seated blockade in the defence of the entire system, hindering self-regulation. 'Effector cells' are hindered by 'suppressor cells'. When two pyramids (inverted cathedrals) occur in the viral and bacterial areas, this may indicate a psychoimmunological phenomenon.*"

If both extracellular and intracellular blockages are present, it initially indicates a trauma that should be investigated. If regulatory T lymphocytes also increase (refer to page 78), immune tolerance is diminished, meaning that pathogenic cells are not recognized and attacked as effectively.

This illustrates how an initially emotional or psychological event can develop into an oncological condition over the years. Micro-Immunotherapy thus offers excellent possibilities for preventing the development of cancer.

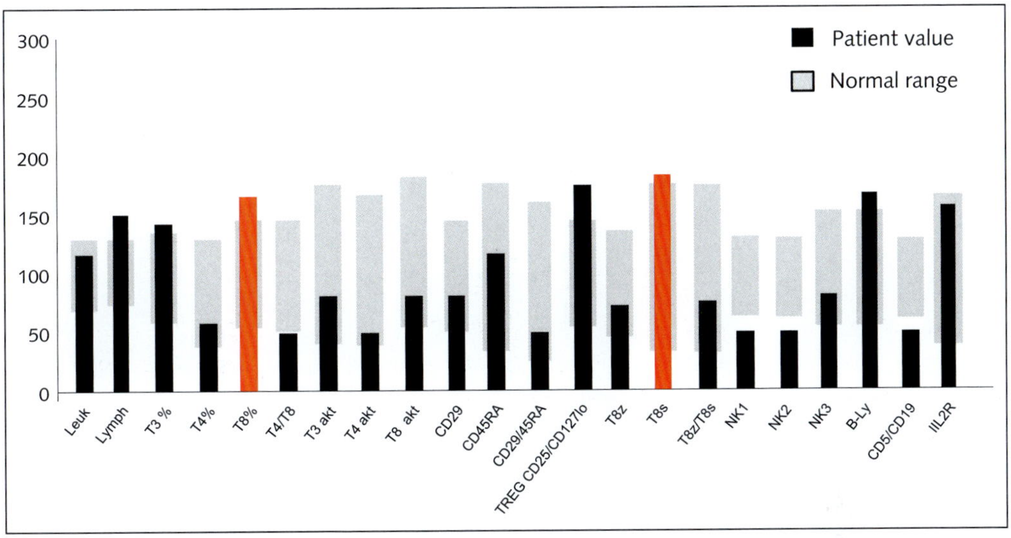

Fig. 27: Rising T8 and T8s Lymphocytes, also called Teeth of Dracula

10 Serum Protein Profile

Another laboratory analysis that Micro-Immunotherapy draws on is the so-called "Serum protein profile".

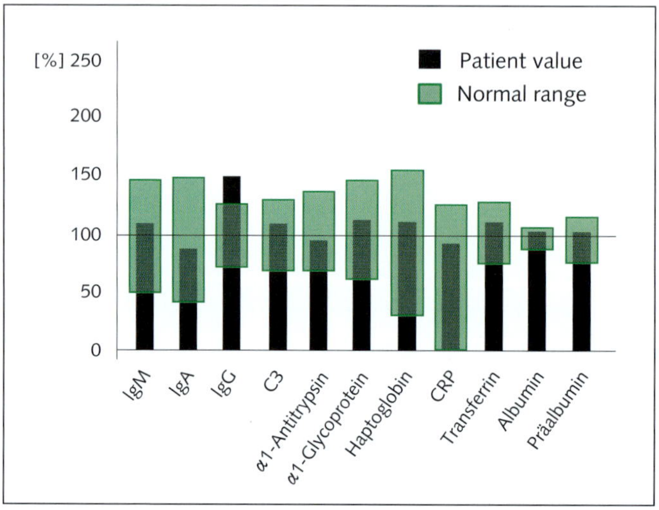

Fig. 28: Serum Protein Profile

▶ Figure 28 shows an example of a patient serum protein profile. The following parameters are determined for this:

- Immunoglobulins IgA, IgM, IgG
- C3 complement,
- Alpha-1 antitrypsin,
- acidic alpha-1-glycoprotein,
- Haptoglobin,
- CRP,
- Transferrin,
- Albumin,
- Prealbumin.

The following guidelines apply to the interpretation of serum protein profiles:

- Immunoglobulins are antibodies.
- They are elevated in subacute or chronic inflammatory diseases and autoimmune diseases. When isolated elevation occurs, it could indicate a monoclonal gammopathy, which might also be associated with a smoldering multiple myeloma.
- Immunoglobulins are reduced in congenital or acquired antibody deficiency, caused by factors such as immunosuppressive therapy, hematological systemic diseases, or renal protein loss.

10.1 Immunoglobulins A (IgA)

Immunoglobulin A (IgA) are antibodies that are primarily found in body secretions, including mucous membranes (intestine), saliva, digestive juices, tear fluid, gastric acid, nasal mucus, lung secretions, and likely synovial fluid (joint lubricant) as well as in breast milk. High concentrations of IgA in breast milk provide protection against vomiting and diarrhoea illnesses in infants.

Increase of IgA in:

- Infections affecting mucous membranes
- Liver damage, liver cirrhosis (especially due to alcohol or other toxins)
- Sarcoidosis
- Crohn's disease
- Rheumatoid arthritis
- Glomerulonephritis
- Plasmacytoma (= multiple myeloma)

Reduction of IgA occurs in immunodeficiency diseases:

a) Primary immunodeficiency (independent disease) is a mostly congenital immunodeficiency.
b) Secondary immunodeficiency is caused by another disease and is therefore much more common than primary immunodeficiency.

Causes can be:

- Malignant tumours
- Leukaemia, lymph node cancer, multiple myeloma
- Medications, such as cortisone and chemotherapy immunosuppressants z. e.g., cyclosporine
- Irradiations
- Protein losses via the intestine
- Protein losses via the kidney - nephrotic syndrome
- Burns (extensive; protein and white blood cells are lost)
- extreme malnutrition

10.2 Immunoglobulins M (IgM)

During a primary infection (initial encounter of the immune system with a pathogen), IgM antibodies are produced first, followed by IgG at a later stage. IgG antibodies remain detectable for a longer period, whereas IgM antibodies tend to decline. This provides us with an indication of whether the infection is recent or not.

Increase in IgM:

- in infections, especially in the acute phase. If IgM remains elevated for a longer period, this may indicate a transition to an active permanent infection (chronic active infection)
- Less frequently in sarcoidosis
- in diseases of the liver (incl. infections)
- Liver cirrhosis, hepatitis in the acute phase
- for lymphatic cancers
- in Waldenström's disease
- In the newborn, an increase in IgM is an indication of a disease in the infant, but IgG comes from the mother

Reduction of IgM in immunodeficiency diseases:

a) Primary congenital immunodeficiency

b) Secondary immunodeficiency is caused by another disease and is therefore much more common than primary immunodeficiency.

Causes can be:

- Malignant tumours
- Leukaemia, lymph node cancer, multiple myeloma
- Medications such as cortisone and chemotherapy immunosuppressants
- Irradiations,
- Protein losses via the intestine
- Protein losses via the kidney – nephrotic syndrome
- Burns (extensive; protein and white blood cells are lost)
- extreme malnutrition

10.3 Immunoglobulins G (IgG)

Immunoglobulins G (IgG) constitute the majority of immunoglobulins because they persist throughout life after an infection, serving as the immune system's antibody memory.

Furthermore, IgG is the only type of antibody that crosses the placenta from the mother to the unborn child, providing protection to the child during the initial weeks of life.

Elevation of IgG in:

- chronic inflammation,
- autoimmune diseases,
- Lymphomas: Hodgkin and non-Hodgkin
- Plasmacytoma (= multiple myeloma)

Reduction of IgG (immunoglobulin G) in immunodeficiency diseases:
a) Primary congenital immunodeficiency
b) Secondary immunodeficiency is caused by another disease and is therefore much more common than primary immunodeficiency.

Causes can be:
- Malignant tumours,
- Leukaemia, lymph node cancer, multiple myeloma,
- Medications, such as cortisone and chemotherapy, immunosuppressants,
- Irradiations,
- Protein losses via the intestine
- Protein losses via the kidney – nephrotic syndrome,
- Burns (extensive; protein and white blood cells are lost),
- extreme malnutrition,
- Viral load, e.g., EBV, measles, rubella.

10.4 C3 Complement

C3 complement is a positive acute-phase protein that belongs to the non-specific immune defence.

It is elevated in acute inflammations and infections.

It is reduced in the case of complement consumption, e.g., in immune complex diseases:
- Glomerulonephritis,
- Systemic Lupus Erythematosus (SLE) and
- in the case of congenital complement deficiency.

10.5 Alpha-1-Antitrypsin

Alpha-1-antitrypsin is also an acute phase protein.

An increase in the alpha-1-antitrypsin level occurs in:
- acute relapses of chronic inflammatory processes,
- Tumours (especially bronchial carcinoma),
- Pregnancy or oestrogen treatment.

A decrease in the alpha-1-antitrypsin level occurs in:
- inherited alpha-1 antitrypsin deficiency,
- Icterus prolongatus or hepatitis of the newborn,
- Cirrhosis of the liver,
- Pulmonary emphysema.

10.6 Alpha-1-Glycoprotein

The acidic alpha-1-glycoprotein (AGP or ORM) is a plasma protein belonging to the fraction of alpha-1 globulins.

Acidic alpha-1-glycoprotein (AGP) is an acute-phase protein present in blood plasma. It constitutes approximately 1 to 3% of the plasma proteins. AGP is mainly produced in hepatocytes and plays a role in the first phase of nonspecific immune defence. Normal plasma levels range between 0.6 and 1.2 mg/ml.

In the plasma, the acidic alpha-1-glycoprotein acts as a transport protein for lipophilic substances. Unlike albumin, it also binds to basic substances such as Propranolol or Lidocaine, with stronger binding observed in men compared to women. During pregnancy, the physiological levels of acidic alpha-1-glycoprotein are reduced.

10.7 Haptoglobin

Haptoglobin is one more acute phase protein.

It is reduced in:
- Intravascular haemolysis,
- congenital haptoglobin deficiency.

It is elevated at:
- acute inflammation.

10.8 C-Reactive Protein (CRP)

CRP is utilized as a non-specific inflammatory marker to assess the severity of inflammatory (bacterial acute) diseases linearly, with higher values indicating greater inflammation. Typically, the CRP concentration in plasma reflects disease activity with a delay of 12 to 24 hours. The expression of CRP is triggered by interleukin 6 (IL-6).

In viral infections, the CRP concentration remains either slightly elevated or not increased at all.

10.9 Transferrin

Transferrin is a glycoprotein that mainly serves to transport iron.

Transferrin is elevated in iron deficiency.

It is reduced in:

- acute inflammation,
- renal protein loss and iron overload
- in liver diseases and liver insufficiency

10.10 Albumin

Albumin serves primarily to maintain colloid osmotic pressure. Albumin is also found in milk, eggs and wheat.

Albumin is reduced in the following conditions:

- Liver synthesis disorders such as liver insufficiency and liver cirrhosis.
- Protein loss syndromes, such as increased loss through the kidneys or the intestines.

Elevated albumin levels are not clinically relevant.

10.11 Prealbumin

Synonyms: transthyretin, thyroxine-binding prealbumin, TBPA, TTR. Prealbumin correlates well with a person's nutritional status.

It is depressed at:

- Tumour diseases,
- Cirrhosis of the liver,
- Protein loss,
- Malabsorption,
- Oestrogen intake,
- Zinc deficiency,
- Malnutrition,
- acute inflammation.

It is elevated at:

- Taking ovulation inhibitors,
- Hypothyroidism,
- Cortisone intake,
- Taking anabolic steroids or androgenic steroids,
- Alcohol poisoning.

10.12 Immunoglobulins E (IgE)

For the detection of allergies, it is advisable to also measure the total IgE levels, as this has significant diagnostic relevance in allergy cases. Elevated IgE levels are also observed in cases of endoparasite infections.

11 HLA Typing

HLA (Human Leukocyte Antigens) are present on the surface of antigen-presenting cells such as dendritic cells and are responsible for distinguishing between self-tissue and foreign substances. If HLA recognizes tissue as foreign, the immune system is activated, particularly T-lymphocytes, which identify and bind to the foreign HLA. As a result, the immune response leads to the rejection of the specific tissue. Researchers discovered HLA during investigations into tissue transplantation. Initially, scientists introduced the English term "MHC" (major histocompatibility complex)[43].

Tissue is recognized and destroyed as foreign when the HLA characteristics of the donor and recipient significantly differ. Under certain circumstances, however, self-tissue may be recognized as foreign, even when the HLA matches, and an immune reaction should not be triggered. The immune system targets and destroys the body's own tissue, leading to autoimmune reactions.

In the recognition of pathogens, antigen-presenting cells also display an HLA characteristic to the immune system, along with an antigen. If the HLA characteristic does not match, i.e., does not correspond, it indicates foreign tissue that needs to be fought against (as seen in transplantation). In the case of intracellular infections, the immune response involves the destruction of infected self-cells with a matching HLA characteristic. The specific HLA type determines how this process occurs. This, too, is an autoimmune reaction.

HLA typing makes it possible to identify autoimmune tendencies because certain HLA characteristics are associated with specific autoimmune diseases. Scientists have already identified several disease-associated HLA markers (refer to table p. 98), and they continue to discover more. However, it's essential to note that while the HLA pattern provides an indication of whether a patient may be at risk for a particular autoimmune disease, HLA typing only determines a relative risk for developing an associated condition and is, therefore, not a definitive diagnostic tool.

43 Since all vertebrates have MHC complexes, the term "HLA" (human leukocyte antigen) was later coined for the human MHC - for the purpose of differentiation.

11.1 Nomenclature

The designation of an HLA[44] is composed of:

- the abbreviation HLA,
- a hyphen,
- one or two letters for the isotype or gene locus (e.g., HLA-B or HLA-DR),
- for class II genes, the letter A or B to identify the gene for the α - or β-chain (e.g., HLA-DRB),
- for class II gene loci with multiple genes,
- a digit (e.g., HLA-DRB3 for the 3rd gene at the HLA-DRB gene locus),
- an asterisk (*) as a separator,
- an allele group number designating the specific antigen variant (e.g., HLA- B*27),
- a colon as a separator,
- a number indicating the variant (allele) of the protein (e.g., HLA-B*15:01),
- another colon as a separator,
- a number indicating a variant with synonymous nucleotide substitution (e.g., HLA-B*15:01:01),
- another colon as a separator,
- a number indicating variants in non-coding sequences (introns) (e.g., HLA-B*15:01:01:02),
- a letter as a suffix coding for abnormalities in expression (see table, e.g., HLA-B*15:01:01:02N for a non-expressed variant).

There are Two Classes of HLA:

1. Class I antigens (subclass Ia: HLA-A, HLA-B, HLA-C; subclass Ib: HLA-E, HLA-F, HLA-G) As of the end of 2105, 10,297 HLA class I alleles are known.
2. Class II antigens (HLA-DM, -DO, -DP, -DQ, -DR) there are 3,543 known HLA class II alleles at the end of 2015.

Class I is presented to the T8c lymphocytes together with an intracellular process (viral, or cancerous). Class II is presented by the antigen-presenting cell to the T4 lymphocytes.

HLA typing is a genetic diagnostic procedure. Anyone who carries out genetic diagnostics must adhere to legal guidelines. In Germany, a new Genetic Diagnostics Act (GenDG) has been in force since 1.2.2010 – the guidelines have been tightened again.

44 Source http://hla.alleles.org/ [retrieved 12.12.2015]

A genetic examination may only be conducted if patients provide written consent. Therapists have a duty to inform, meaning that before the patient gives consent, they must be informed about the nature, purpose, and potential risks of the examination. Furthermore, the law stipulates that patients must be offered appropriate counselling after the examination. Additionally, the law requires that patient samples be destroyed immediately after analysis, but the examination data must be retained for ten years.

However, Micro-Immunotherapy does not use HLA typing for the detection or early detection of diseases and risks. Instead, it employs it to create a therapeutic agent. Therefore, as a therapist, you could have patients sign a waiver. By doing so, patients would waive the explanation of the results and only request the therapy. Since HLA typing only indicates a relative risk of disease development rather than a confirmed illness, you can request HLA typing with a clear conscience. Nevertheless, the therapist should thoroughly inform their patients before conducting the examination. Forms are available at your specialized laboratory.

11.2 HLA Characteristics and Disease Association

There is currently no reliable HLA database since the significance of HLA types varies depending on the ethnic background. Different ethnic groups, such as Africans, Asians, Caucasians, or indigenous tribes, interpret individual HLA characteristics differently. Specialized laboratories exist that, based on previously diagnosed diseases, associate certain HLA types and maintain their own databases. Recently, medical professionals and therapists have been using a patient's HLA characteristics for diagnosing specific diseases. As researchers are expected to identify more disease-associated HLA types in the future, databases are still under development. The following example is therefore incomplete and only applies to white Europeans. It aims to provide a brief insight within this book into how the connections between disease or pathogens and HLA can be interpreted.[45] (Only excerpts from the table in this book are shown).

45 Source: http://www.laborlexikon.ch/Lexikon/Infoframe/h/HLA-Typisierung.htm [retrieved 16.3.2021]

11.3 HLA Table

Disease	HLA Antigen	Relative Risk **
Orthopedics/Rheumatology/Collagenosis		
Ankylosing Spondylitis	B27	Increased 87.4 times
M. Reiter	B27	Increased 37.0 times
Reactive Arthritis:		
Shigella	B27	Increased 20.7 times
Salmonella	B27	Increased 17.6 times
Yersinia	B27	Increased 17.6 times
Gonococci	B27	Increased 13.9 times
Borrelia, Lyme Arthritis, Chronic Form		
>12 months	DR2	Increased 5.0 times
1 - 5 months	DR4	Increased 13.0 times
	DR2+ DR4	Increased 22.0 times
Psoriatic arthritis	B27	Increased 10.7 times
	B38	Increased 9.1 times
Rheumatoid arthritis	DR4	Increased 10.2 times
Juvenile rheumatoid arthritis	DR8	Increased 9.0 times
	DR5	Increased 3.3 times
Lupus erythematosus	DR3	Increased 4.3 times
	B8	Increased 4.6 times
Lupus nephritis	DR2+ DQ1	Increased 14.0 times
Sjögren's syndrome	DR3	Increased 9.7 times
Sarcoidosis	B8	Increased 2.8 times
	B13	Increased 3.1 times
	B8+ B13	Increased 8.5 times
Ophthalmology		
Scleritis	B15	Increased 4.1 times
Acute anterior uveitis	B27	Increased 10.4 times

▶

Disease	HLA Antigen	Relative Risk **
Diabetic retinopathy	B8	Increased 4.0 times
Neurology		
Narcolepsy	DQ6*0602	Increased 130.0 times
Multiple Sclerosis	DR2	Increased 4.1 times
Schizophrenia	A9+ B27	Increased 11.9 times
	A2+ A11	Increased 9.8 times
Myasthenia gravis	A1	Increased 2.6 times
	B8	Increased 3.0 times
	DR3	Increased 2.9 times
	DR5	Increased 2.6 times
M. Alzheimer	B7	Increased 2.8 times
	B7+ Cw3	Increased 28.0 times
Nephrology		
Goodpasture's syndrome	DR2	Increased 15.9 times
Idiopathic membranous glomerulonephritis	DR3	Increased 12.0 times
IgA nephropathy	DR4	Increased 5.5 times
Haematology		
Pernicious anemia	DR5	Increased 5.4 times
Gastroenterology		
Cholelithiasis (gallstones)	A19	Increased 131.0 times
Hepatitis B, chronic course	B35	Increased 158.0 times
Healthy Hbs-Ag carriers	B41	Increased 11.2 times
Chronic active hepatitis	B8+ DR3	Increased 13.9 times
	DQ6*0603	Increased 14.0 times
Haemochromatosis	A3	Increased 6.7 times
	B14	Increased 26.7 times
	A3+ B14	Increased 90.0 times

▶

Disease	HLA Antigen	Relative Risk **
Coeliac disease	B8	Increased 11.0 times
	DR3	Increased 10.8 times
	DR7	Increased 11.9 times
	DR3+ DR7	Increased 52.1 times
	DQ2	Increased 36.4 times
Endocrinology		
Type I diabetes	DR3	Increased 5.8 times
	DR4*0405	Increased 49.0 times
	DQ2	Increased 38.0 times
	DQ3	Increased 22.5 times
	DR5	Increased 0.4 times*
	DR15	0.2 times increased*
	DQ7	Increased 0.1 times
M. Addison	B8	Increased 3.9 times
	DR3	Increased 6.3 times
	DR3	Increased 6.3 times
M. Basedow	B8	Increased 3.3 times
	DR3	Increased 3.2 times
Hashimoto's thyroiditis	DR4	Increased 3.1 times
	DR5	Increased 3.2 times
Subacute Thyroiditis	B35	Increased 13.7 times
Dermatology		
Psoriasis vulgaris	B13	Increased 4.7 times
	B17	Increased 4.7 times
	B37	Increased 6.7 times
	Cw6	Increased 13.3 times
Lichen planus	DR1	Increased 11.8 times
	DQ1	Increased 5.3 times
	A30	0.2 times increased*

▶

Disease	HLA Antigen	Relative Risk **
M. Behçet	B51	Increased 6.3 times
Dermatitis herpetiformis	B8	Increased 8.7 times
	DR3	Increased 15.4 times
Alopecia areata (circular hair loss)	B12	Increased 5.4 times
Gravidity		
Postpartum thyroiditis	DR4	Increased 5.3 times
	DR5	Increased 3.2 times
Atopies		
Aspirin-sensitive asthma	DQ2	Increased 4.1 times
Analgesic asthma syndrome	A1+ B8 + DR3	Increased 5.9 times
Ragwort allergy	B7	Increased 3.6 times
Insulin allergy	B7	Increased 3.3 times

*A relative risk <1.0 means negative association = reduced risk of disease

** Relative risk (RR*) for gene carriers to get the disease compared to non-gene carriers.

HLA is an individual representation of the predisposition to develop a disease. Because it is so unique and individual – a matching HLA is very rarely found – it can explain why the same virus can trigger completely different diseases in different individuals. This circumstance makes it impossible to statistically capture diseases and therapies. By determining the HLA, we can offer a specific therapy tailored to each individual.

As research continues to uncover new connections and gain new insights, it is advisable to stay informed regularly about the current state of research.

With increasing knowledge in genetics and epigenetics, it has been recognized that HLA is not fixed. Therefore, HLA is also referred to as polymorphism, indicating variations rather than genetic defects. For instance, it has been demonstrated that the Epstein-Barr virus can influence HLA in its favor through DNA methylation, especially in oncological conditions such as nasopharyngeal carcinoma, Burkitt's lymphoma, Hodgkin's lymphoma, and others.[46]

All HLA characteristics are always determined and utilized for therapy. In addition to HLA types that may trigger diseases, there are also HLA types that offer protection against diseases. For instance, there exists an HLA characteristic that provides protection against HIV infection and, consequently, AIDS[47]. This particular characteristic was discovered during investigations aimed at understanding why some HIV-infected individuals never develop AIDS or only do so very late in the disease progression. Many therapists are familiar with the fact that HLA-B27 predisposes individuals to diseases like ankylosing spondylitis. However, it is less known that it is also associated with psoriasis.

46 Singh S, Banerjee S. Downregulation of HLA-ABC expression through promoter hypermethylation and downmodulation of MIC-A/B surface expression in LMP2A-positive epithelial carcinoma cell lines. Sci Rep. 2020 Mar 25;10(1):5415. doi: 10.1038/s41598-020-62081-0. PMID: 32214110; PMCID: PMC7096436. [accessed: 13 Mar 2021

47 Cruse JM, Brackin MN, Lewis RE, Meeks W, Nolan R, Brackin B: HLA disease association and protection in HIV infection among African Americans and Caucasians. Source: http://www.ncbi.nlm.nih.gov/pubmed/1910527 [retrieved 13.3.2021].

12 Autoantibodies

"Autoantibodies" refer to antibodies that target the body's own tissues, hormones, or other antibodies. The presence of autoantibodies is an indication of autoimmune diseases.

Autoantibodies can be utilized both for diagnosis and for monitoring therapy.

The following table[48] illustrates autoantibodies and their association with autoimmune diseases.

Autoantibodies	Autoimmune Disease
Acetylcholine receptor antibody	Myasthenia gravis
ANCA (ACPA, granulocyte cytoplasm)	Wegener's granulomatosis vasculitis Ulcerative Colitis Crohn's disease Primary sclerosing cholangitis
AMA (Mitochondria)	PBC (primary biliary cirrhosis) Lues
ANA/ENA antibodies (antinuclear antibodies)	Collagenoses rheumatoid arthritis autoimmune chronic hepatitis type I
Goblet cell antibody	Ulcerative colitis
Colonic epithelium	Ulcerative colitis
ds-DNA antibody (double-stranded DNA)	Lupus erythematosus
Endomysium antibody	Coeliac disease/Sprue's disease Dermatitis herpetiformis
Epidermal basement membrane	Pemphigoid
GADA (Glutamate decarboxylase antibody)	Type 1 diabetes

▶

48 http://www.laborlexikon.ch/Lexikon/Infoframe/a/Autoantikoerper.htm [retrieved 13.3.2021]

- epidermal growth factor (EGF)
- fibroblast growth factor (FGF)
- granulocyte-macrophage colony stimulating factor (GM-CSF)
- hepatocyte growth factor(HGF)
- insulin-like growth factors (IGF)
- Interleukines IL-1β and IL-8
- nerve growth factor (NGF)

The nerve growth factor (NGF) was discovered by Rita Levi-Montalcini. Researchers are still exploring ways to selectively activate and increase NGF in order to potentially heal paralyzed individuals or treat patients with multiple sclerosis (MS). The synthesis of NGF receptors is promoted by IL-1 and IL-6. In the case of MS, there is a deficiency of IL-6, which directly relates to NGF and the disease. IL-1 is an inflammatory factor that is chronically inhibited by anti-inflammatory drugs such as salicylic acid or corticosteroids. Therefore, IL-1 is also partially responsible for reduced nerve regeneration in conditions like Alzheimer's or dementia. Additionally, Alzheimer's disease involves a deficiency of the neurotransmitter substance P.

- platelet derived growth factor (PDGF)
- transforming growth factor (TGF)
- vascular endothelial growth factor (VEGF).

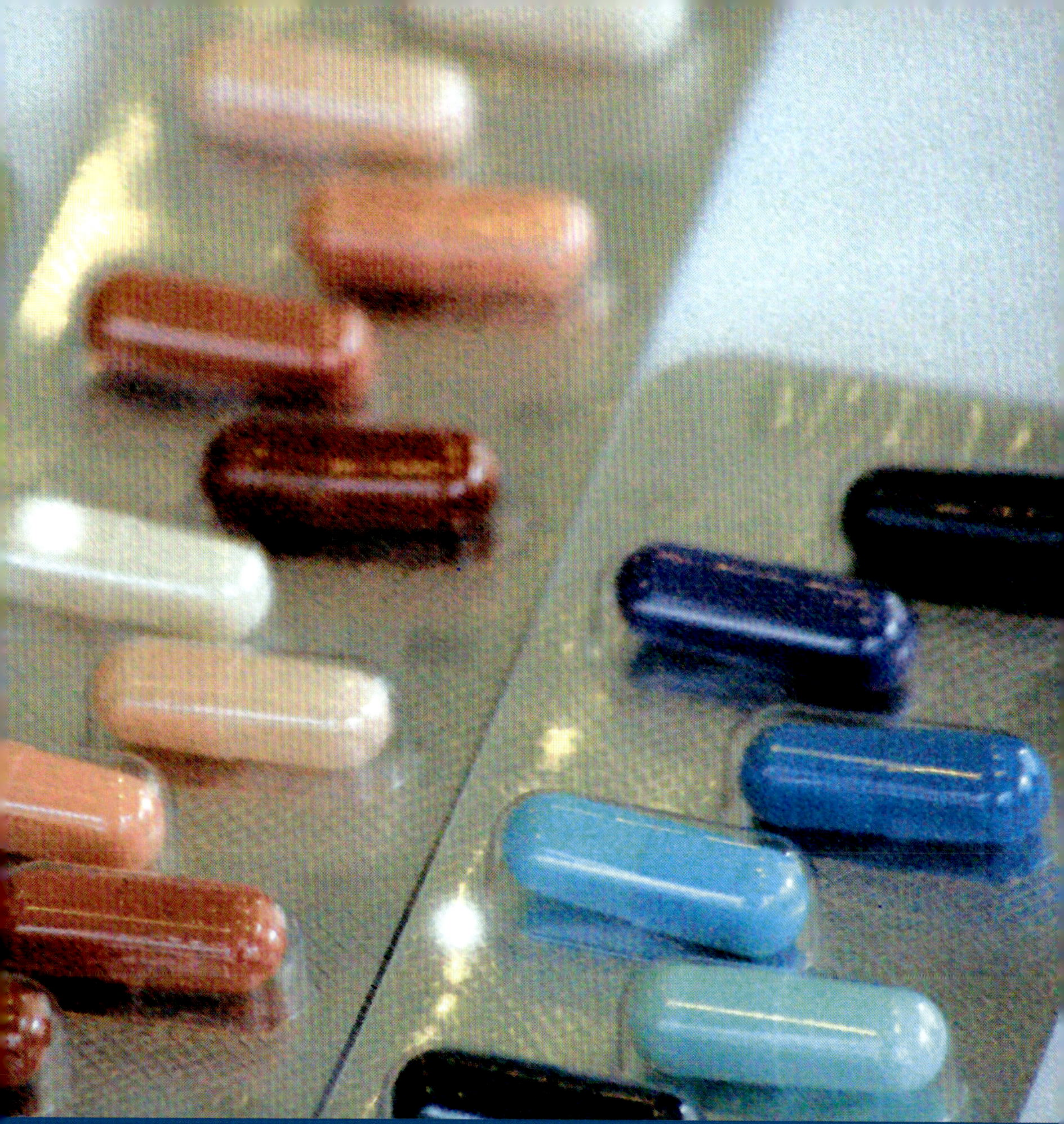

Therapy Setting and Therapy Goals

14 The Treatment

14.1 Therapy Hierarchy

Under no circumstances will it always be feasible to address every discovery stemming from laboratory results.

Firstly the following rule must be observed:

Acute comes before chronic.

As previously stated (refer to Chapter "Serology," p. 48), bacterial and viral parameters testing positive for IgA and/or IgM should be considered as acute events. These should be treated prior to any reactivations, unless: There is a concurrent reactivation of EBV. In such cases, EBV could potentially be causally involved in the event, in a manner where EBV impedes the immune system from ensuring a regular Adaptive defence against acute bacterial and viral infections. Hence, a second rule emerges:

A reactivated EBV must always be treated.

In Micro-Immunotherapy, the assessment of HHV-4: Epstein-Barr Virus (EBV) reactivation is given the highest priority.

If the immune system is weakened, the therapy must be designed to strengthen the immune system, possibly in conjunction with bacterial or viral components.

However, if the immune system is overactive, therapeutic measures to slow it down must be initiated. Furthermore, the cytomegalovirus (CMV) must be considered, as it is very similar to EBV in both clinical manifestation and reactivity.

In Principle, the Following Applies:
Priority should be given to treating what burdens the patient the most, and what has occurred most recently, ahead of what has been present for a long time.

Therapy and Therapy Goals
For the treatment of pathogens not covered by Micro-Immunotherapy products, the use of nosodes is recommended. This will become evident in the practical examples.

▸ *2LARTH*

is a non-specific remedy for arthrosis and arthritis; it can be used without laboratory diagnostics. However, especially in rheumatic conditions, the triggers must be considered for simultaneous treatment. This remedy is also recommended for acute intestinal inflammations.

The intake is carried out for 4 to 6 months, particularly during acute phases. Specific clarification through serology and immune status is advisable. During the acute phase, up to 4 capsules per day are taken.

▸ *2LCHLA*

is a specific remedy for infections with Chlamydia trachomatis and/or Chlamydia pneumoniae (Chlamydophila pneumoniae). This requires serological investigation.

The therapy lasts for 4 to 6 months until serology is under control. It is continued until IgA and/or IgM are confirmed negative.

▸ *2LCMV*

is used as a specific remedy for CMV infections and/or reactivations, both in cases of compromised and normal immune status.

The preparation **2LXFS** (refer to page 125) is indicated for hyperactive immune systems. Treatment is administered for a minimum of 6 months until serological control. Administration can be ceased only when values return to the normal range.

▸ *2LDMLA*

is suitable as a non-specific remedy for the treatment of age-related macular degeneration (AMD). The author has also had very positive experiences with the agent in the treatment of wet macular degeneration.

Administered daily is 1 capsule, until clinical improvement occurs. This could happen as early as a few months. Afterward, the intake is reduced to every other month.

▶ *2LDEP*

is a remedy that can be used for treating depression. It does not require serological investigation. However, depression can also arise from a weakened immune system, so an immune status should be assessed in any case.

Likewise, 2LDEP balances neurotransmitter activity and exerts an influence on the gut-brain stress axis.

▶ *2LEAI*

is used in a hyperactive immune system without EBV, CMV or Toxoplasmosis involvement. Treatment is given for a maximum of 2 months.

▶ *2LEID and 2LEID-N*

2LEID and 2LEID-N are both agents used for a deficient (hyporeactive) immune system. They can and should be administered alongside other specific agents, such as those against EBV, CMV, and herpes.

▶ *2LEID-N*

is an advancement of 2LEID, primarily suitable for acute infections, especially in the field of ENT (Ear, Nose, and Throat) infections, less so for autoimmune conditions.

The typical treatment duration is 2 to 3 months.

▶ *2LEBV*

is a specific remedy for EBV reactivations[54] or chronic mononucleosis, in conjunction with a compromised or normal immune status. In cases of hyperreactive immune systems, 2LXFS (refer to page 125) is the preferred option.

The treatment is conducted for a minimum of 6 months until control is achieved. In some instances, the therapy may extend over 1 to 2 years.

54 Glady, G. and Reigh, L.: Study of the effect of specific Micro-Immunotherapy in patients suffering from chronic diseases associated with Epstein-Barr virus (EBV). Erfahrungsheilkunde, Issue 5 2005, Haug Verlag.

▸ *2LHA*

is suitable for the treatment of hepatitis A. Therapy continues until symptoms cease and liver transaminase levels have normalized.

▸ *2LHC and 2LHCX*

are suitable as specific remedies for hepatitis B and C and D.

▸ *2LHCX*

is administered in the case of a hyperreactive immune system. Here, too, therapies are administered until no more viral copies are detectable by PCR.[55]

▸ *2LHERP*

is suitable as a specific remedy for the treatment of infections with herpes virus types 1 and 2. In acute cases, up to 3 cps. daily may be prescribed.

The duration of therapy is determined by serology; typically, it is carried out for a minimum of 4 months until we control again.

▸ *2LINFLAM*

is used for acute and chronic inflammations, especially during inflammatory flare-ups in autoimmune diseases like Multiple Sclerosis or rheumatic conditions. 2LINFLAM is particularly effective when dealing with elevated CRP levels.

The recommended treatment duration is approximately 2 to 3 months. During acute flare-ups, up to 3 capsules can be taken daily.

▸ *2LMDA*

is a remedy for Alzheimer's disease. The duration of the therapy depends on the symptoms.

---

55 The polymerase chain reaction (PCR) is a technique used to produce numerous copies of specific segments of DNA (deoxyribonucleic acid = the hereditary information-bearing chains in chromosomes). This technique can be employed for the detection of infectious agents such as bacteria and viruses, the identification of genetic disorders, as well as for establishing paternity or identifying perpetrators ('genetic fingerprint').

▶ *2LMEMSENIOR*

is specifically designed for the treatment of older individuals and patients with reduced cognitive function. It is typically administered over several years.

▶ *2LMIREG*

regulates mitochondrial activity, which is often the cause of burnout. It is suitable for patients with impaired mitochondrial activity or genetically induced mitochondrial insufficiency (e.g., deficiency in SOD or detoxification difficulties in the mitochondria). In cases of corresponding genetic predisposition, this treatment should be administered as a long-term therapy over several years.

▶ *2LMISEN*

is a non-specific remedy for stress and aging conditions, as well as the resulting secondary illnesses. It contributes to the activation of atrophic cells and apoptosis. 2LMISEN supports and regulates the immune system in physical or psychological stress situations: In acute situations, take 1 to 2 capsules per day until clinical improvement occurs. For chronic stress: take 1 capsule per day for 2 to 3 months, then 10 capsules per month for an additional 3 to 6 months.

To counteract immune depression caused by stress, 2LEID can be administered simultaneously. The duration of therapy depends on the symptoms.

In order to counteract immunitary depression caused by stress, simultaneously 2LEID can be given.

Duration of therapy according to the symptoms.

▶ *2LOSTEO-N*

This is an extremely interesting and effective remedy for osteoporosis and osteopenia. It primarily contains bone growth factors and silicon. Dentists, for instance, use it to treat patients with bone loss in the jaw area, periodontal disease, and periodontitis. There is an experiential study by a French dentist[56] on OSTEO-N, in which he successfully treated periodontal disease and loose teeth.

Osteopenia often arises from deficiencies in Vitamin D, calcium, and other trace elements, as well as chronic inflammatory processes. Therefore, proper diagnosis and treatment are necessary.

It should be noted that osteoporosis is an autoimmune disease and requires careful micro-immunotherapeutic diagnosis.

The therapy usually lasts 6 months.

▶ *2LPAPI*

is a specific remedy for HPV infection. The decisive factor for using this remedy is the detection of the virus through PCR (see footnote on page 120) in the swab sample.

The treatment duration is at least 4 months until control. Treatment continues until no more Papilloma viruses are detectable.

Often, in patients with an abnormal PAP test, reactivated EBV is also present. It is essential to treat this as well.

▶ Note: The terms "Papillomavirus" and "Pap test" are fundamentally unrelated. The Pap test was developed and introduced by Greek physician George Papanicolaou in 1928. It is based on the evaluation of stained cell samples from the cervix of a woman and serves for the early detection of cervical cancer.

One possible cause for altered cells can be Papilloma viruses. The author's experience has shown that, for example, in Switzerland, pathogen detection is done far too rarely. Often, it is not Papilloma viruses but herpes viruses types 1 and 2 that are found, which are responsible for a poor Pap test (see page 160).

is a specific agent for HPV infection. The decisive factor for the use of this agent is the detection of viruses by PCR (see footnote p. 120) in the smear.

---

56 Jean-Marie Clercq: Growing old - Micro-Immunotherapy applied to periodontal diseases: 2LOSTEON medication, designed to sustain the immune system of patients affected by osteoporosis, seems to be also well adapted to the periodontal disease of jaws.

▶ *2LPARK*

is suitable as a remedy for Parkinson's disease. In this case, micro-immunotherapeutic diagnostics, including serology and immune status assessment, must be carried out initially. Only after potential burdens have been investigated and treated can further therapy with 2LPARK be considered. This remedy also proves effective for treating Restless Legs Syndrome.

A lifelong maintenance therapy is conducted with breaks of 1 to 2 months.

▶ *2LPR*

is the preferred remedy for polyarthritis. However, given that the causes of rheumatic diseases can be diverse and highly variable, thorough diagnostics and appropriate treatment are necessary.

▶ *2LPSO*

is suitable for Psoriasis. Similarly, the patient must undergo micro-immunotherapeutic assessment initially. Once existing burdens have been treated, treatment with 2LPSO can continue.

Therapy is continued until no clinical manifestations remain. It's important in this context to differentially diagnose Psoriasis from Neurodermatitis.

▶ *2LS1 and 2LS2*

are specific remedies suitable for the treatment of HIV infections and AIDS. 2LS1 is used during the acute phase, while 2LS2 is used during stable conditions. The detection of HIV viruses is carried out through RT-PCR[57].

▶ *2LSEN*

is a non-specific remedy primarily designed to support immunity in aging and degenerative processes (Good Aging).

57 In RT-PCR, single-stranded RNA is transcribed into complementary double-stranded DNA using the enzyme reverse transcriptase (RT). This transcript is then amplified with PCR. The RT-PCR method can be used, for example, to detect RNA viruses or to examine expression patterns at the mRNA level.

There are several published studies by Dr. med. Cesare Santi and Dr. med. C. Mor[59], conducted at the outpatient oncology department in Milan. All studies conclude that 2LC1 prolongs survival and significantly improves quality of life. It also enhances the tolerability of chemotherapy and thus its effectiveness.

The therapy is continued until complete tumour remission.

▶ *2LC2*

This is used when no new tumours or metastases have occurred for a duration of 2 years after complete remission of a solid tumour.

The therapy duration is at least 2 years, followed by administering one package every 2 months per quarter.

▶ *2LCL1 and 2LCL2*

These are used for lymphatic cancer types such as Hodgkin's and Non-Hodgkin's lymphomas or hairy cell leukaemia.

Note that these diseases often have a causal connection with HHV-4: Epstein-Barr Virus (EBV).

Therefore, testing for EBV is important and if positive, it should be treated accordingly.

Important control values include the total leukocyte count, lymphocyte count, platelet count, and red blood cell count. Elevated leukocyte and lymphocyte count in a leukaemia patient do not indicate hyperreactivity of the immune system, and thus, this immune status is not controlled with hyperactivity-targeting remedies.

The therapy continues until complete remission.

▶ *2LCL2*

This is administered only after complete remission, typically for at least 2 years. If lymphopenia is present (a deficiency of lymphocytes), it can be treated concurrently with 2LEID or 2LEID-N.

---

59 Micro-Immunotherapy as a complementary cancer therapy: a study with metastatic patients. Journal of Tumour Marker Oncology, Volume 18, Number 2, Spring 2003, The International Academy of Tumour Marker Oncology Inc Publishers.

▶ *2LCLM*

This is the remedy of choice for myeloid leukaemia. Additional therapy for EBV is also indicated.

▶ *2LKAH*

Developed for the treatment of plasmacytoma, also known as multiple myeloma or Kahler's disease. This is a cancer where plasmacytes degenerate and uncontrollably multiply during their formation in the bone marrow.

The disease presents with general and nonspecific symptoms such as fatigue, exhaustion, unintended weight loss, night sweats, and fever. Bone pain, particularly in the spine, is also typical but not specific.

Adaptive defence of EBV as well as herpes viruses types 1 and 2 should be assessed. The therapy continues until complete remission.

▶ *2LLNH1*

Developed for the treatment of non-Hodgkin lymphomas. Similarly, it's important to assess HHV-4: Epstein-Barr Virus (EBV) treat if necessary.

The therapy duration is until complete remission.

▶ *2LTNM*

A relatively new remedy for the treatment of malignant neural tumours, such as brain tumours.

It's administered until complete remission.

14.4 Substances Used as Unitarians

The author expresses a fundamental critique regarding the use of unitarian remedies. This stance is rooted in the belief that employing single remedies lacks a holistic approach. A linear application that doesn't encompass the entirety goes against the fundamental principles of Micro-Immunotherapy. The anticipation of the response from the entire network remains uncertain in such cases.

However, certain remedies can prove highly beneficial when employed judiciously.

Please be aware that the utilization of these substances requires a thorough understanding.

Desoxyribonucleicum Acidum (ADN) 8CH

Ribonucleicum Acidum (ARN) 8CH

The areas of use derive from the properties and dilutions of the components.

They include immune support in pathologies related to immune deficiency.

Bone Morphogenetic Protein-2 5CH

Induces bone and cartilage formation, key role in the differentiation of osteoblasts.

Bone Morphogenetic Protein-4 5CH

Regulates the formation of teeth, bones, and extremities from the mesoderm; facilitates bone fracture repair.

- *Interleukin 1 (IL-1) 4CH*

- *Interleukin 1 (IL-1) 27CH*

They include immune support in immune pathologies related to an increased or decreased expression of interleukin 1 (IL-1 is mainly a proinflammatory Cytokine).

- *Interleukin 2 (IL-2) 4CH*

- *Interleukin 2 (IL-2) 27CH*

They include immune support in immune pathologies related to an increased or decreased expression of interleukin 2. IL-2 helps stimulate the proliferation of T-Lymphocytes, which are important for recognizing and attacking foreign invaders in the body, such as cancer cells.

▶ *Interleukin-6 4CH*

In individuals diagnosed with multiple sclerosis (MS), a deficiency of IL-6 is frequently observed. Paradoxically, IL-6 plays a protective role for the myelin sheaths surrounding nerve cells. Consequently, it is advisable to incorporate a low potency of IL-6 as a standalone component.

▶ *Interleukin-10 30CH*

When dealing with an intense EBV reactivation or chronic mononucleosis, treatment using 2LEBV may induce an EBV crisis. This could result in symptoms such as lymph node swelling, flu-like manifestations, fever, and fatigue. Given that EBV generates a cytokine similar to IL-10, an excess of IL-10 can occur. To mitigate this, a C30 potency, which entails a high dilution, can help slow down the process.

▶ *RANTES 27CH*

RANTES[60] is a chemokine that holds significant relevance in dentistry. Remarkably elevated levels of RANTES have been identified in the jaw bones of individuals afflicted with osteonecrosis[61]. Furthermore, elevated RANTES levels are detected in various systemic inflammatory conditions. These encompass inflammatory rheumatic disorders, allergies, asthma, multiple sclerosis, and certain tumour-related conditions.

14.5 Compatibility

All remedies are generally well-tolerated. Similar to homeopathy, initial aggravations might occur. When treating EBV, EBV crises are possible, which can resemble common flu-like infections.

As the globules are administered sublingually, they usually bypass the digestive tract. Consequently, even patients with lactose intolerance can take the products. Micro-Immunotherapy is successful in treating such intolerances effectively.

60 Another name is CCL5 (CC-chemokine ligand 5).

61 Lechner J., von Baehr V.: RANTES and fibroblast growth factor 2 in jawbone cavitations: triggers for systemic disease? Int J Gen Med. 2013 Apr 22;6:277-90. doi: 10.2147/IJGM.S43852. Print 2013 http://www.ncbi.nlm.nih.gov/pubmed/23637551 [accessed: 16 Mar 2021].

Compatibility With Other Methods

Micro-Immunotherapy can be combined with all holistic methods, especially classical homeopathy, which aids in treating both symptoms and constitution.

14.6 Nosode Preparations

Nosode therapy and isopathy are crucial complementary approaches to Micro-Immunotherapy. The therapeutic principle aligns with that of Micro-Immunotherapy, encompassing treating like with like. Furthermore, nosode therapy addresses pathogens for which Micro-Immunotherapy does not provide comprehensive remedies.

The selection of nosode preparations or isopathic treatments is at the discretion of each therapist.

14.7 Other Methods

Ideal complements also include all detoxification methods, phytotherapy, manual therapies, and energy work. Energy work, in particular, is highly effective for chronic illnesses as many patients suffer from energy depletion due to persistent pain, fatigue, infections, or allergies.

Further Meaningful Measures

It's always beneficial to conduct source investigations. Particularly, foci of infection in the dental area, as well as structural changes, contribute to chronic diseases by up to 50 percent. Therefore, when treating, it is essential to examine the teeth and address potential sources of infection.

▸ *Orthomolecular Therapy*

Recognizing and treating deficiencies in nutrients, vitamins, and trace elements is crucial.

▸ *Mitochondrial Therapy*

Investigating nitrosamine stress and mitochondrial functionality is advisable, along with relevant supplementary treatment.

15 Clinical Conditions and Selected Cases from Practice

15.1 Attention Deficit/Hyperactivity Disorder (ADHD)

Attention Deficit/Hyperactivity Disorder (ADHD), also referred to as Attention Deficit/ Hyperactivity Syndrome or Hyperkinetic Disorder (HKD), belongs to the group of behavioural and emotional disorders with onset in childhood and adolescence (according to ICD-10: F90–F98, see Table). It is characterized by difficulties in attention, self-regulation, impulsivity, and sometimes marked physical restlessness (hyperactivity).

There are numerous theories regarding the causes of these conditions, if one may even label them as "disorders." Some children undoubtedly struggle simply with the expectation of sitting still in school. Not all children can do that, but it is not an illness!

Classification According to ICD-10[62]

F90.–	Hyperkinetic disorders
F90.0	Simple hyperkinetic disorder
F90.1	Hyperkinetic disorder of social behaviour
F90.8	Other hyperkinetic disorders
F90.9	Hyperkinetic disorder, unspecified
F98.–	Other behavioural and emotional disorders with onset usually occurring in childhood and adolescence
F98.8	Other specified behavioural and emotional disorders with onset usually occurring in childhood and adolescence – Attention disorder without hyperactivity

Among others, the following causal relationships are discussed:

- Emotional, verbal and/or physical violence
- Pressure to perform and stress
- increased sugar consumption
- Food additives
- too much television and online games
- Vaccinations
- poor parental care and attention.

62 ICD-10 online (WHO version 2016) http://www.dimdi.de/static/de/klassi/icd-10-who/kodesuche/onlinefassungen/htmlamtl2016/index.htm [retrieved 3.3.2016]

In September 2010, we encountered a well-adjusted young individual who had resumed engaging in some physical activity. While not entirely recovered, he was motivated to make up for missed schooling.

His HHV-4: Epstein-Barr Virus (EBV) values align with his reported symptoms:

	Date 16.7.2009	Date 16.3.2010	Date 1.9.2010	Reference value
EBV EA IgG IF	**40**	**20**	**<20**	Titer < 20
EBV VCA IgG IF	320	640	320	Titer < 80
EBV VCA IgM IF	<10	<10	<10	Titer < 10
EBV EBNA-1 IgG IF	**<20**	**<20**	**20**	Titer < 20

- EBV early antigen IgG is now absent, with a value of <20.
- EBV VCA IgG has decreased to 320 (previously 640), aligning with the expected pattern (4 times the reference value) for a resolved EBV infection.
- EBV EBNA-1 IgG registers as positive, with a value of 20, confirming the resolution of the EBV infection.

It wasn't until 2015 that we had another encounter with the same patient. On this occasion, he appeared notably pale and expressed feelings of illness. He had successfully completed his A-levels and was currently pursuing studies in computer science, involving prolonged computer usage, complemented by some physical activity.

Given the circumstances, the possibility of HHV-4: Epstein-Barr Virus (EBV) reactivation was evident. Thus, our initial step was to examine his EBV values:

	Date 1.9.2010	Date 21.10.2015	Reference value
EBV EA IgG IF	**40**	**20**	Titer < 20
EBV VCA IgG IF	320	320	Titer < 80
EBV VCA IgM IF	<10	<10	Titer < 10
EBV EBNA-1 IgG IF	20	20	Titer < 20

Indeed, EBV EA IgG showed positive again, corresponding to reactivation of EBV.

Considering the pronounced paleness, we also assessed the levels of vitamin D:

	Date 21.10.2015	Reference value	Explanation
Vitamin D, 25-OH	19	75 – 220 nmol/l	Deficiency 30 – 75 nmol/L
			High deficiency < 30

He was once again administered 2LEBV along with 10,000 I.U.[65] of vitamin D3 and vitamin K2 for a duration of 3 months.

Following another consultation at the end of December 2015, the patient's condition had significantly improved.

This case serves to emphasize an important point:

Frequently, patients visit our clinic feeling entirely unwell, fatigued, and perpetually drained. Many arrive with extensive folders containing numerous abnormal laboratory test results. They often undergo numerous therapies, but even after months, progress remains minimal or absent.

In many instances, investigating the Epstein-Barr virus often uncovers the underlying cause. Nonetheless, both patients and their physicians can find it challenging to accept. Can HHV-4: Epstein-Barr Virus (EBV) alone truly be responsible for such severe symptoms?

Years of experience in our practice have demonstrated that indeed, this can be the case. Of course, any nutritional deficiencies must be identified and treated (e.g., with orthomolecular medicine). However, EBV reactivation, for instance, is consistently implicated in up to 80% of chronic illnesses. Without addressing EBV, symptoms tend to persist. Chronic illnesses also influence mental well-being, making it essential to complement long-term therapies with other approaches.

Providing patients with thorough care is paramount. Reassurance is often sought, confirming that no other issues are present. Given the sometimes bewildering information from the internet and social media, therapists may find it challenging to provide this assurance. For both patients and therapists, cultivating patience is vital.

65 I.U. = International Units

When doctors inform patients that everyone carries EBV and that it's not the root cause of their condition, even if the doctor doesn't have a definitive diagnosis, it doesn't serve anyone well. While the statement that almost 90% of the European population has EBV is accurate, it doesn't negate the possibility of EBV contributing to specific health concerns.

The values for a completely normal HHV-4: Epstein-Barr Virus (EBV) look as follows:

		Reference value
EBV EA IgG IF	<20	Titer <20
EBV VCA IgG IF	320	Titer <80
EBV VCA IgM IF	<10	Titer <10
EBV EBNA-1 IgG IF	80	Titer <20

15.4 Epilepsy

A remarkably compelling case involved a 3-year-old girl.

Her ordeal began when she was merely two years old, experiencing severe epileptic seizures following a combination vaccination for measles, mumps, and rubella (MMR vaccination). Desperate for help, the father sought assistance from our clinic. Comprehensive diagnostic tests were conducted, revealing an unexpectedly negative result for EBV. It's worth noting that a previous patient with epilepsy had visited our practice; their epileptic episodes were attributed to EBV and resolved completely after Micro-Immunotherapy, a resolution still maintained today, even 12 years later.

During discussions, the father presented an extensive folder containing various laboratory results, including a correct EBV analysis that demonstrated a positive EBV VCA IgG and negative EBV EBNA IgG. Remarkably, this critical distinction had gone unnoticed. In essence:

When initially analysed in a hospital setting, prior to cortisone treatment, the child tested positive for EBV with a negative EBV EBNA IgG. This signifies that persistent EBV was already present at the onset of the disease.

The young girl underwent 2LEBV therapy for a span of 2 months. The frequency of her seizures began to diminish, and EBV VCA IgG was once again detected in her serum.

After an additional 6 months of therapy, she experienced a seizure-free existence for the first time. Another 6 months later, the child was able to return to kindergarten.

15.5 Crohn's Disease (CD) and Ulcerative Colitis (UC)

Crohn's disease (CD) is a chronic inflammatory disorder that primarily affects the entire gastrointestinal tract, with a predilection for the colon or the distal small intestine, or sometimes both. Inflammation tends to occur within the deep layers of the intestinal mucosa, typically forming localized foci. This condition may involve regional lymph nodes. The disease tends to progress in episodes, during which fever and a pronounced sense of illness can manifest. Weight loss is also a common occurrence.

Extraintestinal symptoms encompass various manifestations, including aphthae, arthritis, uveitis, and erythema nodosum. These symptoms can provide insights into potential causative agents: for instance, aphthae are frequently associated with herpes simplex, while arthritis can be linked to Yersinia enterocolitica infection.

Genetic factors have been described in the context of MC, involving chromosomes 14 and 16, as well as the influence of six HLA alleles. These genetic factors can exert either a negative or positive influence.

Negative genetic factors include:
- HLA-DR1
- DQ5 and DR13 in Caucasian populations
- HLA-DR7 in the French and German populations
- HLA-DR4 and DQ4 in the Japanese population.

A positive effect of HLA DR3 is also under suspicion.

Similar to previously mentioned viruses and bacteria, potential triggers include those mentioned here as well. In the case of bacteria, particularly those that colonize the intestinal mucosa are of interest, distinguishing it from ulcerative colitis, which tends to affect the mucosal surface. Both Crohn's disease and ulcerative colitis have higher prevalence rates in Northern Europe and North America. Medical experts estimate an annual occurrence of 4 to 6 new cases per 100,000 inhabitants. Italian researchers have highlighted a significant correlation between high carbohydrate consumption in MC and UC patients and their consumption of fast food.

In clinical practice, I've frequently observed the involvement of parasites or herpes simplex viruses 1 and 2 in Crohn's disease cases. Allergic and toxic causes can also contribute, necessitating diagnosis and treatment. It's important to consider a differential diagnosis with celiac disease.

Among immunosuppressed individuals, reactivation of cytomegalovirus can lead to what's termed "CMV colitis."

Yersinia enterocolitica is among the most common pathogens linked to Crohn's disease (refer to page 19). Additionally, Listeria and Salmonella have been proposed as potential causes. These pathogens all exhibit resistance to cold conditions, leading to a hypothesis that the introduction of cold chains in the food industry could have contributed to the increased incidence of Crohn's disease and ulcerative colitis[66].

Yersinia Enterocolitica

The primary symptom is diarrhoea, which is often caused by colitis, enterocolitis, or terminal ileitis[67]. This symptom can persist for 1–2 weeks, and in some cases, it may extend for several months. Pseudo appendicitis, characterized by symptoms resembling appendicitis such as right lower abdominal pain, can also occur. Enlarged lymph nodes in the abdominal region are a typical finding. Endoscopy reveals signs of ulcerative colitis or Crohn's disease. Reactive arthritis and erythema nodosum are frequently observed. Yersinia-induced myocarditis (carditis) can lead to arrhythmias. Other rare associated conditions may include urethritis, glomerulonephritis, conjunctivitis, or uveitis (Reiter's syndrome).

Treatment

Intestinal disorders are often linked to the environment. In managing chronic inflammations within the digestive tract, it is crucial to maintain a healthy intestinal microbiota.

Chronic intestinal inflammations respond well to treatment with 2LMICI. For acute inflammation, a recommended course of action is 2LARTH for one week, with a dosage of 3 capsules daily.

---

66 Hugot J.P.: Crohn's disease: the cold chain hypothesis, http://dx.doi.org/10.1016/S0140-6736(03)15024- 6 [retrieved: 16.3.2021].

67 Kato Y., Hattori T., Oh-Ya H., Yoshino S., Kato H.: Acute terminal ileitis and Yersinia enterocolitica infection. Gastroenterol Jpn. 1977;12(1):36-43. http://www.ncbi.nlm.nih.gov/pubmed/863177 [accessed 16 Mar 2021].

Practical Example

A patient, born in 1983, presented at our practice in 2014 with a confirmed diagnosis of M. Crohn's disease. The patient expressed a desire to discontinue cortisone treatment.

Immunological analysis revealed a pronounced immune system response, accompanied by a significant reduction in regulatory T lymphocytes (Treg), indicative of an ongoing chronic autoimmune process (refer to page 77 for more information). Additionally, there was a marked increase in NK lymphocytes.

Furthermore, the patient exhibited the following biomarkers:
- Elevated levels of IgA in the serum, pointing towards inflammation within mucous membranes (specifically, the intestine).
- Vitamin D deficiency.
- Reactivation of the Epstein-Barr virus HHV-4: Epstein-Barr Virus (EBV).
- Positive test result for Yersinia infection.

Laboratory results from May 14, 2014, indicated:
- Yersinia enterocolitica IgG: 26 U/mL (reference range: <20 U/mL)
- Yersinia enterocolitica IgA: 54 U/mL (reference range: <20 U/mL)

The treatment plan encompassed the following interventions:
Implementation of probiotic therapy (given the frequent reduction of lactobacilli and coli bacilli in cases of yersiniosis).
Administration of 2LMICI Micro-Immunotherapy to address intestinal inflammation.
Utilization of 2LEBV therapy.
Introduction of Astaxanthin, known for its anti-inflammatory and radical scavenging properties.
Prescription of a daily dose of Vitamin D3 at 5000 I.U.

Remarkably, within just 4 months of initiating treatment (without cortisone), the patient reported significant improvement in his overall well-being. A follow-up evaluation conducted by a gastroenterologist revealed persistent inflammation in the terminal ileum, consistent with yersiniosis. The therapeutic regimen was sustained until the Yersinia IgA antibodies were no longer detectable, which spanned a duration of 12 months.

In the case of ulcerative colitis (UC), the chronic inflammation is confined to the mucous membrane of the colon, usually originating from the rectum and gradually extending distally. The disease is characterized by a pattern of alternating acute flare-ups and symptom-free periods. Unlike Crohn's disease, blood in the stool is more frequently observed in ulcerative colitis. The mucosal surface is more prominently affected.

15.6 Hashimoto's Disease (Autoimmune Thyroiditis)

This autoimmune thyroid disorder is commonly associated with hypothyroidism.

The patient, born in 1967, initially visited our practice in June 2013, presenting with severe neurodermatitis that affected her entire body. Notably, the face and hands exhibited open sores, accompanied by intense itching.

A summarized medical history is outlined as follows:

- Pre-existing Hashimoto's disease, Additional diagnoses: severe neurodermatitis, asthma
- Mother of three children, including a set of twins
- Experienced mononucleosis (EBV) at 18 years old
- Contracted chickenpox at 27 years old
- Dental history: dental restoration completed, retained amalgam fillings, and dental crowns composed of gold, as well as titanium implants.

Laboratory diagnostics from 12.6.2013:

	Pat. Value	Reference Value
EBV EA IgG IF	<20	Titer <20
EBV VCA IgG IF	<80	Titer <80
EBV VCA IgM IF	<10	Titer <10
EBV EBNA-1 IgG IF	<20	Titer <20
Vitamin D, 25-OH	**70**	mmol/l 75-220
T4 free	13,2	pmol/L 10.0-19.8
T3 free	3,2	pmol/L 3.1-6.5
TSH	1,59	mU/L 0.35-4.5
TG (Thyroglobulin) AB	**200**	kIU/L <60
TPO (Thyroperoxidase) AB	**1930**	kIU/L <60
Herpes simplex (HSV) IgG	Pos.	Pos.

	Pat. Value	Reference Value
Herpes simplex (HSV) IF IgM	<20	Titer <20
Herpes simplex (HSV) IF IgA	**80**	Titer <20
Varicella-Zoster (VZV) IF IgG	320	Titer <20
Varicella-Zoster (VZV) IF IgM	<20	Titer <20
Varicella-Zoster (VZV) IF IgA	**80**	Titer <20
Immunoglobulins E	**1265**	kIU/L <114

Cytomegalovirus exhibited slight reactivation, and IgA testing revealed a positive result for Yersinia enterocolitica.

Interestingly, it's worth noting that while EBV testing appears negative, there were previous indications of mononucleosis.

Herpes simplex virus types 1 and 2 have demonstrated a robust positive response in IgA testing, reaching a level of 80. This suggests reactivation. Similarly, there is a positive IgA response indicating reactivation of the varicella-zoster virus.

The patient also presents with a vitamin D deficiency, and although the thyroid gland functions within normal parameters (euthyroid[68]), there is an elevation in autoantibodies. Notably, an allergic predisposition is evident, characterized by markedly elevated IgE levels. Despite conducting allergy tests for airborne allergens (pollen, house dust, etc.) and dietary factors, no conclusive results were obtained.

This combination of positive results for herpes simplex viruses type 1 and 2, reactivated varicella-zoster virus, and elevated IgE levels aligns with a characteristic pattern often observed in neurodermatitis cases in the author's clinical practice.

Lymphocyte Typing

This pertains to a diminished immune condition. The total lymphocyte count is lowered, with activated lymphocytes standing out proportionally. Meanwhile, in the viral defense mechanism, there is an appearance of a pyramid T8c/T8s, which signifies an indication of immune incompetence.

68 exhibiting normal thyroid function

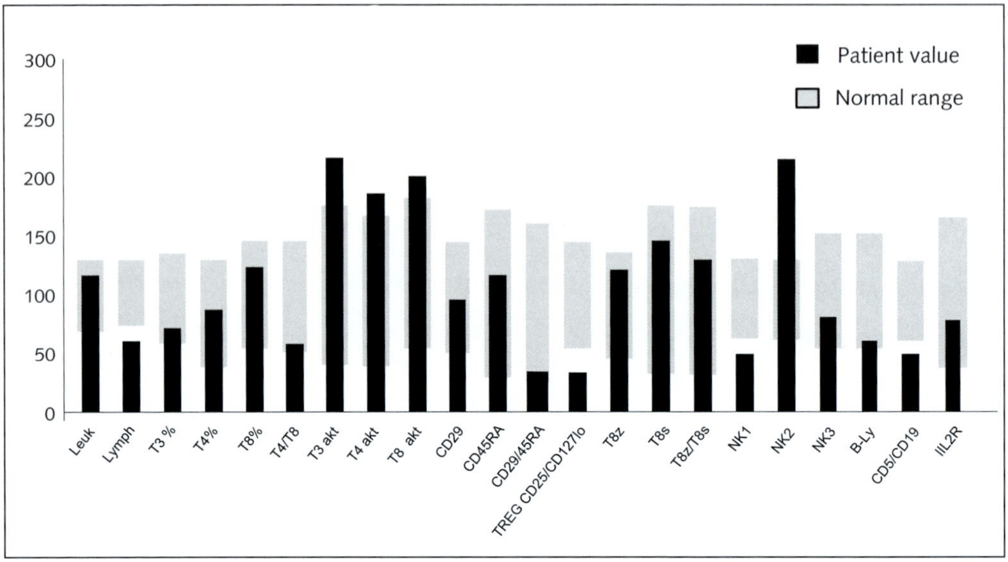

Fig. 29: Lymphocyte Typing of the Patient

Therapy

- 2LZONA
- 2LHERP
- 2LALERG

- Neythymun No. 29 f + k pro Inject. St. II Amp.1x per week
- Vitamin D3 5000 I.U. plus K2 daily.

After 5 months of therapy, a new laboratory assessment was conducted to either validate the ongoing treatment or consider an alternative strategy.

	Pat. Value 6/2013	Pat. Value 11/2013	Reference Value
EBV EA IgG IF	<20	<20	Titer <20
EBV VCA IgG IF	<80	320	Titer <80
EBV VCA IgM IF	<10	<10	Titer <10
EBV EBNA-1 IgG IF	<20	80	Titer <20
Vitamin D, 25-OH	70	113	mmol/l 75-220
T4 free	13,2	–	pmol/L 10.0-19.8
T3 free	3,2	–	pmol/L 3.1-6.5
TSH	1,59	–	mU/L 0.35-4.5

	Pat. Value 6/2013	Pat. Value 11/2013	Reference Value
TG (Thyreoglobulin) Ak	200	–	kIU/L <60
TPO (Thyroperoxidase) Ak	1930	–	kIU/L <60
Herpes simplex (HSV) IgG	Pos.	Pos.	Pos.
Herpes simplex (HSV) IF IgM	<20	<20	Titer <20
Herpes simplex (HSV) IF IgA	80	80	Titer <20
Varicella-Zoster (VZV) IF IgG	320	320	Titer <20
Varicella-Zoster (VZV) IF IgM	<20	<20	Titer <20
Varicella-Zoster (VZV) IF IgA	80	20	Titer <20
Immunoglobulins E	1265	1760	kIU/L <114

It's immediately noticeable that EBV now appears as having been overcome. This indicates that EBV has an immunological relevance in this condition and requires therapeutic attention. Varicella-zoster activity has subsided with an IgA level of 20, yet herpes simplex remains reactivated. Vitamin D levels have now normalized.

Although the patient did experience some improvement in well-being and skin condition, the skin remained quite dry.

The subsequent treatment plan was as follows:

- 2LEBV
- 2LHERP
- 2LALERG
- Borage oil capsules, 500 mg, taken 3 times daily (to address dry skin)
- Neythymun No. 29 f + k, administered via injection, St. II Amp, once weekly
- Vitamin D3, 2000 I.U. daily

A follow-up assessment was scheduled after 6 months, with a blood sample planned for May 2014. However, during this time, the patient reported experiencing hair loss, intense itching, and profound exhaustion. The neurodermatitis had entered an acute flare-up, causing the patient considerable distress.

The lab results are as follows:

	Pat. value 6/2013	Pat. value 11/2013	Pat. value 5/2014	Reference value
EBV EA IgG IF	<20	<20	<20	Titer <20
EBV VCA IgG IF	<80	320	320	Titer <80
EBV VCA IgM IF	<10	<10	<10	Titer <10
EBV EBNA-1 IgG IF	<20	80	80	Titer <20
Vitamin D, 25-OH	**70**	113	**54**	mmol/l 75–220
Ferritin	101		**24**	µg/L 30–300
T4 free	13,2	–	10,3	pmol/L 10.0–19.8
T3 free	3,2	–	3,6	pmol/L 3.1–6.5
TSH	1,59	–	1,2	mU/L 0.35–4.5
TG (Thyroglobulin) Ak	200	–		kIU/L <60
TPO (Thyroperoxidase) Ak	1930	–		kIU/L <60
Herpes simplex (HSV) IgG	Pos.	Pos.	Pos.	Pos.
Herpes simplex (HSV) IF IgM	<20	<20	<20	Titer <20
Herpes simplex (HSV) IF IgA	**80**	**80**	**40**	Titer <20
Varicella-Zoster (VZV) IF IgG	320	320	–	Titer <20
Varicella-Zoster (VZV) IF IgM	<20	<20	–	Titer <20
Varicella-Zoster (VZV) IF IgA	**80**	20	–	Titer <20
Immunoglobulins E	**1265**	**1760**	**1054**	kIU/L <114

Assessment

- Ferritin is significantly low
- Vitamin D remains in the deficient range
- Total lymphocytes are also reduced (not shown in the table)

Therapy and Treatment Goal:
While the deterioration in the patient's condition can be supported by the laboratory results, aside from iron deficiency and Vitamin D deficiency, which could contribute to hair loss, the values are not entirely explainable. This might indicate an underlying disruptive factor, often found to be dental in origin, specifically within the teeth. The significantly elevated IgE allergy marker could also suggest this possibility.

As a result, a computer-regulated thermography was initiated. The results indicated the presence of significant dental disturbances, particularly with the gold crowns and titanium implants, along with high toxic exposure. Further investigations with a dentist and laboratory analysis using the Lymphocyte Transfer Test for titanium and gold revealed that the gold crowns needed to be replaced due to intolerances. Fortunately, no titanium intolerance was detected, allowing the implants to remain.

This was followed by a detoxification therapy and extensive dental treatment, including replacing the gold crowns and bridges.

Therapy
- Vitamin D 3 10'000 I.U. daily
- Vitamin K2
- Coral Calcium
- Stoffwechsel Eisen Dr. Töth (Life Light)
- IgE C30
- Borage Oil Kps 3 x 500 mg to be continued
- 2LEBV, 2LHERP omitted, because so far not responding to therapy
- Base powder from Dr. Töth
- Spirulina Iron from Life Light
- Detox therapy

A subsequent assessment took place after 4 months, revealing the following outcomes:
- Ferritin levels were within the normal range
- Vitamin D3 levels had normalized
- Total lymphocyte count had decreased
- The patient reported feeling notably weak, although there was an improvement in skin condition

Further Therapy

- 2LEBV
- 2LEID for 2 months
- Vitamin D3 still 2000 I.U. daily
- L-lysine 2 x 500 mg daily
- NADH 5 mg in the morning
- Borage Oil Cps. still 3x 500 mg
- Astaxanthin 4 mg daily
- If the persistent itching becomes intolerable, it was considered to use an antihistamine for relief.

A larger follow-up examination took place in August 2015:

	Pat. Value 6/2013	Pat. Value 11/2013	Pat. Value 5/2014	Reference Value
EBV EA IgG IF	<20	<20	<20	Titer <20
EBV VCA IgG IF	<80	320	640	Titer <80
EBV VCA IgM IF	<10	<10	<10	Titer <10
EBV EBNA-1 IgG IF	<20	80	80	Titer <20
Vitamin D, 25-OH	**70**	**54**	**61**	mmol/l 75–220
Ferritin	101	**24**	60	µg/L 30–300
T4 free	13,2	–	10,3	pmol/L 10.0–19.8
T3 free	3,2	–	3,6	pmol/L 3.1–6.5
TSH	1,59	–	0,92	mU/L 0.35–4.5
TG (Thyroglobulin) Ak	**200**	**–**	**134**	kIU/L <60
TPO (Thyroperoxidase) Ak	**1930**	**–**	**977**	kIU/L <60
Herpes simplex (HSV) IgG	Pos.	Pos.	Pos.	Pos.
Herpes simplex (HSV) IF IgM	<20	<20	<20	Titer <20
Herpes simplex (HSV) IF IgA	**80**	**40**	**40**	Titer <20

	Pat. Value 6/2013	Pat. Value 11/2013	Pat. Value 5/2014	Reference Value
Varicella-Zoster (VZV) IF IgG	320	–	320	Titer <20
Varicella-Zoster (VZV) IF IgM	**<20**	–	<20	Titer <20
Varicella-Zoster (VZV) IF IgA	**80**	–	**20**	Titer <20
Immunoglobulins E	1265	2481	1054	kIU/L <114

After over two years of therapy, the patient's condition has significantly improved, a fact supported by vastly improved laboratory results. Nonetheless, the journey is not entirely complete:

- HHV-4: Epstein-Barr Virus (EBV) has risen and now appears to be reactivated
- Herpes simplex viruses types 1 and 2 remain reactivated, as indicated by positive IgA results
- While autoimmune thyroid antibodies have decreased, they are still present
- A pronounced allergic predisposition still exists, though less severe compared to the beginning of the treatment

The Ongoing Therapy Plan Includes:

- 2LHERP
- 2LEBV
- 2LALERG
- Daily intake of Vitamin D, 2000 I.U.
- L-Lysine, 3 times daily at 500 mg each
- Continued use of Borage oil capsules, 3 times daily at 500 mg each

This case demonstrates that Micro-Immunotherapy can be effective in treating complex autoimmune conditions, making the disease more manageable. Furthermore, it highlights the need for multiple approaches to address complex diseases and emphasizes the necessity for patience, both on the patient's part and that of the therapist. It's likely that another two years will be required for all symptoms to vanish, and setbacks are to be expected along the way.

15.7 Multiple Sclerosis

In Multiple Sclerosis (MS), chronic inflammatory processes primarily affect the brain or the spinal cord. This disease involves the destruction of the myelin sheaths surrounding nerve cells. MS is an autoimmune disorder, often post-infectious in nature, and its development is influenced by genetic predisposition. The emergence of MS typically involves three key components:

- Genetic disposition.
- Agents that trigger inflammation in the brain or spinal cord.
- A toxic element capable of breaching the blood-brain barrier.

A strong genetic predisposition is evident:
HLA-DR2 and HLA-DQ2, as well as HLA-DR3, commonly associated with HLA-A1 and HLA-B8, and less frequently with HLA-A3 and -B7.
As potential triggers, primarily "neurotropic" (nerve-attacking) agents are considered, alongside any factors that can lead to autoimmune processes.

This includes:

- the entire family of Herpes viruses,
- especially Epstein-Barr Virus HHV-4: Epstein-Barr Virus (EBV)[69],
- Varicella Zoster,
- Measles,
- Tick-borne Encephalitis virus,
- Polio viruses,
- Cytomegalovirus,
- Adenoviruses,
- Canine distemper virus CDV (Canine Distemper)[70],
- and JC Virus[71] (Human Polyomavirus 2).

The extent to which chronic toxic burden in the oral region could be responsible for the disruption of the blood-brain barrier has unfortunately never been investigated. However, this does seem to fall within the realm of possibility. Highly toxic metals such as mercury, silver, and tin can indeed penetrate the central nervous system.

Some researchers have also established a connection between MS and the presence of destructive fatty acids. Specific substances, such as arachidonic acid, have been identi-

69 Ascherio, A., MD, DrPH and Munger, K.L., MSc , Environmental risk factors for multiple sclerosis. Part I: The role of infection, Annals of Neurology 19 APR 2007 http://dx.doi.org/10.1002/ana.21117 [retrieved 16.3.2021].

70 Hodge, M.J., MD, PhD and Wolfson, C., PhD Canine distemper virus and multiple sclerosis, Neurology August 1997 vol. 49 no. 2 Suppl 2 S62-S69 http://dx.doi.org/10.1212/WNL.49.2_Suppl_2.S62 [retrieved 16.3.2021]

71 In connection with the intake of Tysabri®, MS patients who carry the JC virus are advised not to take the drug over a longer period of time because encephalitis could occur. The question is, of course, to what extent the JC virus could be causally involved in the development of MS?

fied to actively promote inflammation. It effectively serves as the driving force behind the inflammatory process.

Arachidonic acid originates from linoleic acid found in food. Individuals with inflammatory degenerative conditions like MS or rheumatism are advised to follow a diet low in linoleic acid to mitigate the potential exacerbation of their symptoms.

The progression of the disease typically occurs in episodes, showcasing symptoms such as:

- Sensory disturbances and motor weaknesses,
- Inflammation of the optic nerve,
- Dysfunction of the bladder sphincter,
- Speech disorders.

Treatment approaches vary according to each case, but the following principles generally apply:

- Detoxification therapy and rebalancing of the body's environment,
- Addressing individual viral or bacterial loads,
- Micro-Immunotherapy tailored to immune status and serology,
- Micro-Immunotherapy offers the product 2LSEP.

The body's own nerve regeneration factors such as transforming growth factor (TGF-ß), ciliary neurotrophic factor (CNTF) and glial cell-line derived neurotrophic factor (GDNF) support the restoration of the myelin sheaths. These substances are available in homeopathic dilution

▶ Summary

Multiple Sclerosis (MS) is a multifactorial disorder. Its development requires a convergence of various triggers that interact. It is well-established that heavy metals like mercury in amalgam fillings can disrupt the blood-brain barrier. A prominent German manufacturer of amalgam, involved in a highly publicized lawsuit with an MS patient organization, made a significant payment without being pronounced guilty. Nonetheless, since then, the company ceased the production of amalgam. Mercury is also found in vaccines. Consequently, vaccines could potentially contribute to the disruption of the blood-brain barrier, enabling viral agents to penetrate the brain. For instance, measles, polio, or tick-borne encephalitis (TBE) viruses are frequently detectable even in the cerebrospinal fluid of MS patients.

Two factors play a crucial role in the development of MS: the presence of triggers and the presence of MS-associated HLA markers.

Beyond the pathogens mentioned earlier, neurotropic agents are also implicated in causing MS, primarily Epstein-Barr Virus (EBV). Scientific research has confirmed the significant role of HHV-4: Epstein-Barr Virus (EBV) in MS. It is presumed that similar mechanisms are at play in all autoimmune diseases, contingent on the HLA markers.

The notion that external factors contribute to the immune system's attack on the myelin sheaths within the brain and spinal cord, leading to MS, is not new. EBV has long been considered among the prime suspects. Recent insights have revealed that in MS patients, the jugular veins collapse. This leads to constrictions, even complete stenoses, impeding the proper drainage of blood from brain areas. Circulating viral or bacterial agents remain in the brain for extended periods. This phenomenon also results in pressure differentials, potentially compressing brain areas. These changes, encompassed by the term "chronic cerebro-spinal venous insufficiency" (CCSVI)[72], are currently a topic of contention within MS research.

15.8 Neurodermatitis

In our practice, we encounter numerous cases of neurodermatitis. These cases share several common features:

- Adaptive defence of Epstein-Barr Virus (EBV),
- Reactivation of Herpes simplex,
- and/or Varicella Zoster.
- In some cases, an allergic component is evident, while in others, an inflammatory aspect is present, and frequently, both occur simultaneously.
- The immune status is typically compromised in both the viral and bacterial defense mechanisms.

The following example illustrates the case of a 17-year-old young woman. She is still attending school and is a high-level athlete.

72 Zamboni P, Galeotti R, Menegatti E, Malagoni AM, Tacconi G, Dall'Ara S, Bartolomei I, and Salvi F: Chronic cerebrospinal venous insufficiency in patients with multiple sclerosis. Journal of Neurology, Neurosurgery, and Psychiatry. 2009 Apr; 80(4): 392-9.

Serology

	March 2002	Reference value
EBV EA IgG IF	<20	Titer <20
EBV VCA IgG IF	1280	Titer <80
EBV VCA IgM IF	<10	Titer <10
EBV EBNA-1 IgG IF	40	Titer <20
Herpes 1 and 2 IgG	640	Titer <20
Herpes 1 and 2 IgM	<20	Titer <20
Herpes 1 and 2 IgA	80	Titer <20
Varicella Zoster IgG	320	Titer <20
Varicella Zoster IgM	<20	Titer <20
Varicella Zoster IgA	160	Titer <20
IgA total	210	g/l <80
IgE total	324	kIU/Lit <114

In the serology, the reactivated HHV-4: Epstein-Barr Virus (EBV) immediately draws attention. Additionally, there are IgA-positive values for Herpes Virus Type 1 and 2, as well as for Varicella Zoster.

Also noteworthy is the presence of both inflammatory and allergic diathesis, evident in the significantly elevated levels of total IgA and total IgE.

Lymphocyte Typing

In 2002, a graphic of the immune status was not yet available. Elevated T3- and T8-lymphocytes were observed, while T4-lymphocytes were reduced. This pattern corresponds to a pyramid in the bacterial realm. Moreover, the cytotoxic T8-lymphocytes were diminished in relation to T8s, forming a second pyramid in the viral domain.

Two pyramids suggest a psychological component. As a competitive ski racer, the patient faced immense performance pressure, and neurodermatitis meant the end of her athletic career as she could no longer comfortably wear the tight racing suits.

By the time of the first edition of this book, a decade had passed since the case occurred, and the patient had not experienced any further complaints. Remarkably, it was she who suggested the idea of writing this book!

In 2010, she returned to our practice.

From her initial recovery until 2010, she had remained free of neurodermatitis. However, after a significant fall from a climbing wall in 2010, she sustained fractures in two lumbar vertebrae, necessitating a replacement in the first surgical intervention and fixation in a subsequent surgery.

Approximately one week following the second surgery, her neurodermatitis resurfaced.

Immune Status

A closer examination of her immune system[73] revealed a pyramid pattern in the extracellular defence (T4, T8) and a staircase pattern in the intracellular defence (T8c, T8s). This particular configuration can be interpreted as an expression of the trauma she had experienced. In the aftermath of the accident, it wasn't immediately evident whether she had incurred lasting damage

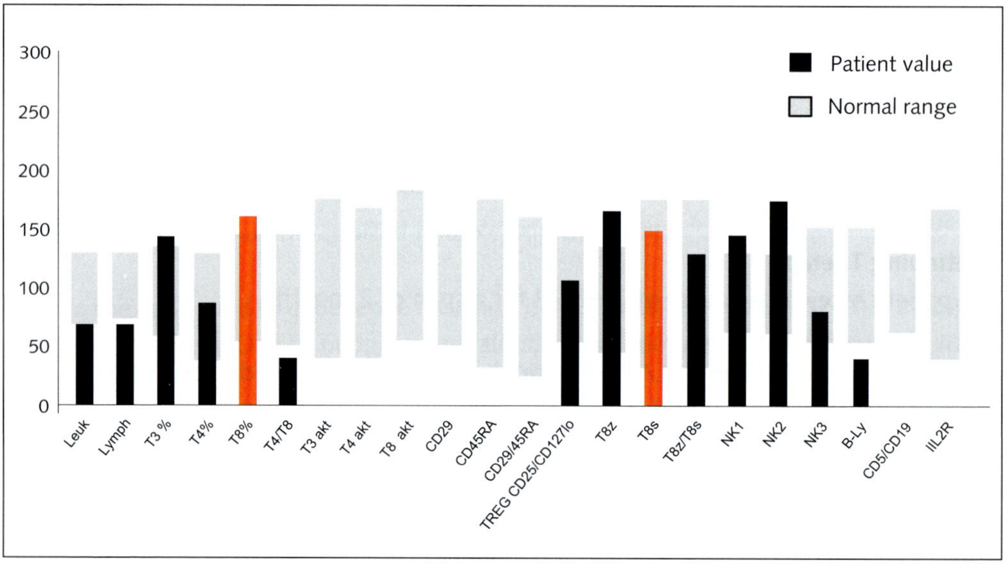

Fig. 30: Lymphocyte Typing of the Patient

73 The findings date back to 2010, at that time not all values in the lymphocyte typing were done, therefore some values do not appear.

Serology

	March 2002	Sept. 2002	July 2010	Reference value
EBV EA IgG IF	<20	<20	<20	Titer <20
EBV VCA IgG IF	**1280**	320	160	Titer <80
EBV VCA IgM IF	<10	<10	<10	Titer <10
EBV EBNA-1 IgG IF	40	80	20	Titer <20
Herpes 1 and 2 IgG	**640**	160	**640**	Titer <20
Herpes 1 and 2 IgM	<20	<20	<20	Titer <20
Herpes 1 and 2 IgA	**80**	**40**	**80**	Titer <20
Varicella Zoster IgG	320	80	160	Titer <20
Varicella Zoster IgM	<20	<20	<20	Titer <20
Varicella Zoster IgA	**160**	**20**	**<20**	Titer <20
IgA total	**210**	**110**	**193**	g/l <80
IgE total	**324**	**160**	**324**	kIU/Lit <114

The impact of reactivation due to trauma is evident in the following observations:

- HHV-4: Epstein-Barr Virus (EBV) levels are notably low overall, suggesting an insufficiency in antibody numbers. It's possible that EBV is hindering the immune response.
- Herpes simplex viruses 1 and 2 have been reactivated with IgA positivity.
- Both IgA and IgE total levels are significantly elevated once more.

Treatment Approach:

- Over a span of 2 months: 2LEID and 2LEBV
- Subsequently, for an additional 4 months: 2LHERP and 2LALERG

Following this regimen, the patient once again became completely symptom-free. By August 2013, she had given birth to a healthy child.

15.9 Pap Smear and Human Papilloma Virus (HPV)

Regrettably, confusion often arises due to terminology. The term "Pap smear" does not have an initial association with papillomavirus, despite common misconceptions.

Dr. George Papanicolaou, a Greek physician, developed the Pap test in 1928. This screening method involves examining stained cell smears obtained from the cervix of a woman. Its primary purpose is the early detection of cervical cancer.

The test results are divided into the following categories:

Pap I	Normal findings, unremarkable
Pap II	Slight changes visible
Pap III	Unclear or doubtful findings
Pap IIID	Dysplasia findings, cell changes
Pap IV	Immediate preliminary stages of cervical carcinoma
Pap V	Cervical carcinoma

Some of the Papillomaviruses (high risk) are indeed among the potential causes of cervical cancer.

In the author's practice, it has been observed that HHV-1: herpes simplex virus type 1 (HSV-1) and HHV-2: herpes simplex virus type 2 (HSV-2) infections have a higher frequency of contributing to adverse Pap test outcomes than papillomaviruses. This underscores the complexity of the factors influencing cervical health and the various viruses that can impact it.

Treatment for Pap II-IV

1. A concerning Pap test result often indicates a reactivation of Epstein-Barr virus (EBV) in the background. Therefore, it is essential to investigate and clarify the presence of HHV-4: Epstein-Barr Virus (EBV) in the blood serum. Subsequently, appropriate treatment, such as therapy with 2LEBV, should be considered.
2. If herpes simplex viruses types 1 and 2 (HSV-1 and HSV-2) are detected, either in the smear or in the serum, it's important to address these infections as well. Treatment options like 2LHERP should be considered in such cases.

3. In the case of papillomavirus infection, it's crucial to identify their presence in the genital area to initiate targeted treatment. This can also be achieved through a smear test. However, for accurate virus detection, a polymerase chain reaction (PCR) analysis (refer to footnote on page 120) is necessary. Additionally, it's advisable to conduct tests for other viruses, such as herpes viruses, simultaneously

It's worth noting that there are various types of papillomaviruses, categorized into risk groups based on their level of relevance to the development of cervical cancer. These distinctions emphasize the diverse nature of papillomavirus strains and their potential health implications.

The types are:

- "Low-risk" viruses
  HPV 6 and 11 belong to this group and are known as the main cause of warts in the genital area (condylomata acuminata, also called "genital warts"). Other low- risk types are 40, 42, 43, 44, 54, 61, 70, 72, 81 and CP6108.
- "High-risk" viruses
  HPV 16, 18, 31 and 33, but also 35, 39, 45, 51, 52, 56, 58, 59, 68, 73 and 82.
  In almost every occurrence of cervical carcinoma, at least one of the high-risk HPV group can be detected in an HPV screening. Additionally, some cancer conditions in the anal and oral regions are considered to be associated with HPV.
- Possibly "high-risk" viruses
  These include HPV 26, 53 and 66.
- Viruses without clear risk assignment (HPV genotypes of undetermined risk)

In the presence of papillomaviruses, treatment is carried out using 2LPAPI. A study on the application and effectiveness of 2LPAPI is available[74]. The duration of treatment depends on the results of the smear test, and a follow-up HPV PCR test must also be conducted to monitor the therapy's progress.

74 Thomas G., Cluzel H., Lafon J., Bruhwyler J. and Lejeune B.: Efficacy of 2LPAPI®, a Micro-Immunotherapy Drug, in Patients with High-Risk Papillomavirus Genital InfectionAdvances in Infectious Diseases, 2016, 6, 7-14 Published Online March 2016 in SciRes. http://www.scirp.org/journal/aid http://dx.doi.org/10.4236/aid.2016.61002 [accessed 2.6.2016].

16 Micro-Immunotherapy for Cancer

The diagnosis of "cancer" triggers panic in most people. Therefore, discussing cancer is not an easy topic, neither in practice nor in this book. Therapists are required to maintain a neutral stance, as it is not permissible to dissuade individuals from conventional cancer therapy. This is not necessary when patients come with the explicit wish that they do not desire further conventional medical measures.

Cancer is a highly complex ailment with the potential for various components contributing to its development. Within this book, only the micro-immunotherapeutic aspects of cancer can be addressed.

16.1 Solid Tumours

As a general rule, a solid tumour should be surgically removed to prevent its spread. Furthermore, cancer-promoting factors from the environment and diet should be ideally eliminated and avoided. Cancer always signifies cell degeneration. The degenerated cells are either not recognized by the immune system and can divide unchecked, or the immune system is weakened to the extent that it can inadequately destroy the defective cells. This leads to uncontrolled cell growth and the formation of tumours. Cancer doesn't infiltrate cells from the outside; rather, it is a process that develops within the cells.

Causes can be:

- Radiation, especially radioactivity,
- toxic substances in the environment and food,
- Medication, tobacco and alcohol consumption,
- Stress, psychological strain, loss of a positive lifestyle,
- chronic infections,
- chronic inflammation,
- natural ageing of cells.

The causality of chronic infections is of paramount importance to the micro- immunotherapy. Several studies (references[75] and[76]) clearly indicate that at least 6 human viruses, which integrate into DNA, pose a cancer risk and are involved in 10-15% of all cancer cases worldwide.

These are:

- HHV-4: Epstein-Barr Virus (EBV),
- Hepatitis B virus (HBV),
- Hepatitis C virus (HCV),
- Human papilloma virus (HPV),
- Human lymphotropic T-cell virus (HTLV-1),
- The Kaposi's sarcoma associated virus (KSHV).

The mechanisms through which these viruses contribute to carcinogenesis are highly intricate. In some cases, apoptosis is hindered, or cell division is expedited, allowing virus-infected cells to proliferate unnoticed and at an accelerated pace.

Practical Experience with Cancer

The following frequently observed correlations between pathogens or noxious agents and carcinogenesis result from practical experience:

- *Brain tumours,* particularly in children, appear to be influenced by the JC virus[77]. Conversely, there is evidence suggesting that glioblastomas are less common in patients who have had chickenpox compared to those who have never experienced chickenpox[78].

- *Carcinomas of the mouth and throat as well as cancer of the* larynx predominantly arise due to toxic substances. The main causes are alcohol and tobacco abuse.

75 Martin D; Gutkind JS.: Human tumour-associated viruses and new insights into the molecular mechanisms of cancer. Oncogene. 2008 Dec; 27 Suppl 2: S31-42. doi: 10.1038/onc.2009.351. http://www.ncbi.nlm.nih.gov/pubmed/19956178 [accessed 16 Mar 2021].

76 White M.K., Pagano J.S., Khalili K. Clin Microbiol Rev. 2014 Jul;27(3):463-81. doi: 10.1128/CMR.00124-13. Viruses and human cancers: a long road of discovery of molecular paradigms. http://www.ncbi.nlm.nih.gov/pubmed/24982317 [accessed 16 Mar 2021].

77 Okamoto H., Mineta T., Ueda S., Nakahara Y., Shiraishi T., Tamiya T., Tabuchi K.: Detection of JC virus DNA sequences in brain tumors in pediatric patients. http://www.ncbi.nlm.nih.gov/pubmed/15881753 [retrieved: 16.3.2021].

78 Amirian, E.S., et al: History of chickenpox in glioma risk: a report from the glioma international case-control study (GICC), Article first published online: 13 MAR 2016, DOI: 10.1002/cam4.682 [retrieved 16.3.2021].

- *Thyroid cancer* is primarily caused by radioactive radiation, and a potential cause could also be iodine deficiency (leading to goiter formation). Furthermore, the author observes the reactivation of EBV and herpes simplex viruses in many cases.

- *Lung cancer and small cell bronchial carcinoma are* are primarily linked to tobacco consumption, but they are also associated with occupational diseases such as asbestosis, psittacosis[79], as well as chronic asthma caused by the inhalation of toxic substances or fine particles, such as flour dust in bakers, for example.

- *Breast cancer* is unfortunately often associated with the use of oral contraceptives. Hormones from the environment, such as plasticizers found in drinking water, can also have carcinogenic effects. Regarding cyst formation, Adaptive defence is primarily implicated. Therefore, this virus can also be considered partially responsible for breast cancer development. There's also a connection between breast cancer and chronic inflammations in the jawbone. "Simultaneously high levels of CCL5/RANTES and breast cancer metastases were observed in tissue samples of jawbone osteopathies"[80].

- *Cancer in the gastrointestinal tract* can be associated with Helicobacter pylori infection. Diet plays a significant role in this regard. Factors like caffeine and similar substances (such as nicotine) should not be underestimated; they can irritate the stomach lining and lead to chronic gastritis. Colorectal cancer can result from the misuse of laxatives or chronic inflammatory conditions like celiac disease, Crohn's disease, and ulcerative colitis. There's a suspected link to the papillomavirus. The consumption of foods rich in nitrates e.g. sausages, etc. also increases the risk of cancer.

- The development of *pancreatic cancer* is favoured by chronic pancreatitis and diabetes. Nicotine abuse, obesity and vitamin D deficiency are also risk factors.

- *Cancer in the urogenital tract* can be promoted by chronic bacterial and viral inflammations that ascend from lower parts of the tract. These notably include papillomaviruses, herpes simplex viruses 1 and 2, Chlamydia trachomatis, and Yersinia enterocolitica.

---

79 Chlymydiaphila psittaci inhaled through bird droppings, especially in animal keepers and pigeon breeders.

80 Lechner J., von Baehr V.: Hyperactivated signal transduction cascades of the chemokine RANTES/CCL5 in osteopathies of the jawbone in breast carcinoma. German Journal of Oncology 2013; 45: 105-111 http://www.deguz. de/files/DEGUZ/photo/article/Deutsche_Zeitschrift_fuer_Onkologie_Lechner_vBaehr.pdf [retrieved 16.3.2021].

- Cervical cancer frequently arises in association with specific papillomaviruses[81], as well as herpes simplex viruses 1 and 2. Similarly, prostate cancer is commonly linked to herpes simplex viruses 1 and 2, often stemming from chronic prostatitis. This can also be induced, for instance, by activities like cycling or wearing excessively tight trousers.

Therapy

A causal cancer therapy encompasses the following components:

- Elimination of environmental stressors,
- Combatting oncogenic viruses,
- Reinforcement of the immune system,
- Assessment of life circumstances and guidance, along with potential therapeutic measures fostering healthy psychological hygiene.

Micro-Immunotherapy offers suitable agents for these purposes, those addressing viral burdens and those designed for cancer therapies.

- Typically, treatment with 2LC1 or 2LC1-N[82] is administered for 2 years until complete tumor remission, followed by 2LC2 for an additional 2 years.
- For brain tumors, the agent 2LTNM has been developed and is prescribed until complete remission is achieved.
- To enhance the immune system, 2LEID and 2LEID-N are recommended. Monitoring total lymphocyte counts is crucial here, and treatment should be continued only as long as they remain below the normal range.

Micro-Immunotherapy has the means to do this. Those that treat viral strains and those that were developed for cancer therapies.

- As a rule, 2LC1 or 2LC1-N (refer to page 125) is given for 2 years until complete remission of the tumour, then 2LC2 for another 2 years.
- For brain tumours, the drug 2LTNM was developed, which is also prescribed until complete remission.
- 2LEID and 2LEID-N are suitable for strengthening the immune system. Here it is important to check the total lymphocytes again and again and to continue therapy only as long as they are below the norm.

81 So-called "high risk" papilloma viruses are in particular HPV 16: 50 %, HPV 18: 20 %, as well as 31 and 33, but also 35, 39, 45, 51, 52, 56, 58, 59, 68, 73 and 82.

82 In the author's practice, 2LC1 and 2LC1-N are prescribed alternately in blisters (= 10 days).

Therapy Control

The monitoring of cancer should be conducted regularly at intervals that align with therapeutic considerations. The specific measures to be implemented vary depending on the type of cancer and can only be provided as general guidelines:

The follow-up for cancer should take place regularly at intervals that make therapeutic sense. The following measures can be taken - these depend on the type of cancer and can only be listed as a guideline:

- Control of tumour markers
- Lymphocyte typing
- Hemogram (I complete blood count (CBC) or full blood count)
- diagnostic imaging (ultrasound, CT, MRI).

16.2 Leukaemias and Lymphomas

The diagnosis of various leukaemias and lymphomas typically involves lymphocyte typing, bone marrow aspirations, and/or biopsies of affected lymph nodes in the case of lymphomas.

The primary types of leukaemia include:

- Acute Myeloid Leukaemia (AML)
- Chronic Myeloid Leukaemia (CML)
- Acute Lymphoblastic Leukaemia (ALL)
- Chronic Lymphocytic Leukaemia (CLL), which is classified as a low-grade non-Hodgkin lymphoma. If the leukaemia originates from prolymphocytes, it's referred to as Prolymphocytic Leukaemia (PLL) due to its notably more aggressive course compared to CLL.
- Hairy Cell Leukaemia (HCL) is also linked to CLL, where the leukaemia arises from highly developed lymphocyte precursors. The hair-like cytoplasmic extensions of the leukaemia cells give the condition its name.

Possible causes can include:

- Radioactivity
- High-voltage power lines
- Smoking
- Viruses: Human T-cell Leukaemia Viruses (HTLV) I and II pose an elevated risk for certain types of leukaemia. Epstein-Barr Virus (EBV) is also a potential trigger for specific forms of leukaemia.

Micro-Immunotherapy

- For lymphocytic leukaemia, 2LCL1 is administered for 2-3 years or until complete remission, followed by 2LCL2 for another 2 years.
- For myeloid leukaemia, 2LCLM is administered.
- Any potential exposure to EBV (reactivation) should be treated with 2LEBV in addition to the agents for leukaemia.

Lymphomas

- Malignant lymphomas are cancerous growths that originate from the monoclonal proliferation of lymphatic cells. Lymphatic cells are present in lymph nodes, tonsils, spleen, and bone marrow (stem cells).
- The WHO classification distinguishes between Hodgkin lymphoma (formerly known as lymphogranulomatosis) and non-Hodgkin lymphomas. The latter are further categorized into B-cell lymphomas and T-cell lymphomas.

Causes

Based on numerous research findings, the HHV-4: Epstein-Barr Virus (EBV) environmental factors, including glyphosate, are being investigated as potential triggers for both Hodgkin's and non-Hodgkin's lymphomas. "In twenty-six cancer studies involving individuals exposed to glyphosate formulations, the majority indicated no significant correlation. Among these studies, nine focused on non-Hodgkin's lymphoma. Four case-control studies collectively demonstrated an association between the cancer and the herbicide, as did two other comparative studies. The more rigorous investigations accounted for additional exposure to different pesticides and still upheld the connection. This association grew stronger with prolonged exposure to glyphosate. While certain confounding variables and biases couldn't be entirely ruled out, the conclusion is that a connection between glyphosate formulations and non-Hodgkin's lymphoma exists in humans, though causality could only be partially established."[83]

Micro-Immunotherapy

In the case of Hodgkin's lymphoma, the primary therapy involves 2LEBV and 2LCL1 for 2-3 years or until achieving complete remission, followed by 2LCL2 for an additional 2 years.

83 Portier C.; Researchers for environmental health in (In "Horizons" No. 108 March 2016, magazine of the Swiss National Fund for the Promotion of Scientific Research) http://www.snf.ch/de/fokusForschung/newsroom/Seiten/ news-160325-horizons-controversial-is-glyphosate-carcinogenic.aspx [retrieved:24.4.2016]

For non-Hodgkin's lymphoma, treatment entails 2LLNH1.

Multiple Myeloma (Plasmacytoma) M. Kahler

Precisely speaking, multiple myeloma falls under the category of B-cell non-Hodgkin's lymphoma. It involves the abnormal proliferation of malignant plasmacytes responsible for producing antibodies.

The following types are distinguished according to the antibody formed:

- IgG plasmacytoma
- IgA plasmacytoma
- Light chain plasmacytoma (Bence Jones plasmacytoma/light chain disease)
  - κ-chain plasmacytoma
  - λ-chain plasmacytoma

The malignant antibodies induce bone decalcification. Consequently, initial laboratory indications encompass elevated serum calcium levels and signs of anemia.

An assessment of the severity of the condition is determined by:

- The level of protein content,
- The number of lesions in the bones,
- The quantity of plasma cells in the bone marrow,
- The presence of Bence-Jones protein in the urine,
- Reduced levels of IgG, IgA.

The following stages are distinguished:

- Stage I β2-Microglobulin value <3.5 ; Albumin > 3.5
- Stage II C-Value < 3.5; Albumin <3.5 oder β2-Microglobulin 3.5–5.5
- Stage III β2-Microglobulin value >5.5

Micro-Immunotherapy
Primarily, the involvement of EBV must be assessed and treated.

The remedy for multiple myeloma is 2LKAH, derived from Kahler's disease. It is administered until values normalize.

For treatment monitoring, the following are particularly suitable:

- Serum calcium levels,
- β2-Microglobulin,
- Serum Protein profile,
- Immunofixation,
- Imaging assessment of bone lesions.

16.3 Note on Cancer Treatment

In practice, there's often a question about whether Micro-Immunotherapy can cure cancer. The author's extensive experience has shown that there are indeed cases where complete healing occurs. This is typically the situation when patients start therapy very early. Often, it's sufficient to eliminate tumours and commence Micro-Immunotherapy immediately. However, when patients come to us completely exhausted after years of chemotherapy, the prospects are less favourable, as cancer and the treatments have already inflicted significant damage.

Like any other therapy, Micro-Immunotherapy cannot perform miracles. Nevertheless, it's crucial to comprehend that Micro-Immunotherapy can contribute to gaining valuable quality of life. When faced with the decision of living possibly six months with debilitating treatments and a diminished quality of life versus three months with good quality of life and the ability to enjoy daily life at home, those three months are preferable to the six. Ultimately, the patient must make the decision.

Treating cancer requires not only expertise but also ethical guidance. Recommending an 87-year-old woman with breast cancer, who is otherwise in excellent health, to undergo chemotherapy followed by radiation is unethical. It's possible that she could live another 2 years without discomfort through non-conventional medical treatments. In such a case, to administer Micro-Immunotherapy is certainly appropriate.

Afterword

There are numerous diseases that I could present here, ranging from amyotrophic lateral sclerosis (ALS) to type I and II diabetes, hay fever, psoriasis, vasculitis, hepatitis, glomerulonephritis, myasthenia gravis, sarcoidosis, Sjögren's syndrome, and all the other autoimmune diseases, as well as celiac disease or acute cytomegalovirus in pregnancy. There's a wide array of different conditions, scarcely any of which I haven't encountered in practice, and for which there isn't an official therapeutic approach.

However, it's important to note that we don't treat diseases or laboratory results; we treat individuals.

I would like to take this moment to express my gratitude to the many individuals who have visited our practice. It's your experiences that have motivated me to continuously seek more knowledge, explore new therapeutic avenues, and never give up, offering you hope.

This book would not have come to fruition without your presence and inspiration. Thank you!

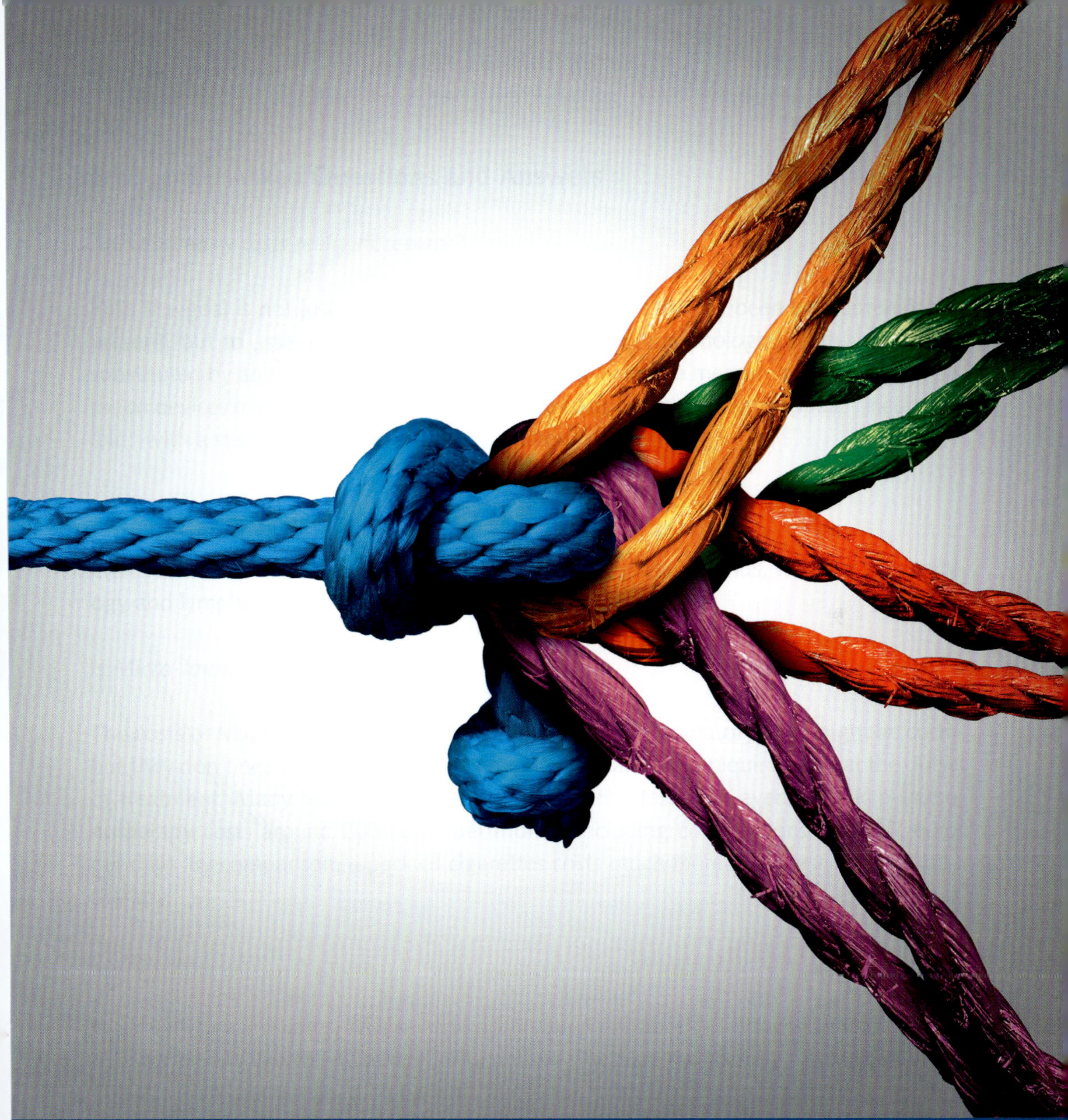

Appendix

Where do the utilized cytokines come from?

The cytokines in Micro-Immunotherapy are cultivated on non-pathogenic E. coli bacteria, making them neither of animal nor human origin.

Why can this therapy be used for so many diseases?

Micro-Immunotherapy's underlying theory posits an infectious-associated cause for all autoimmune diseases. Hence, the therapy can be employed for all autoimmune disorders and other pathologies linked to the immune system. Moreover, there are numerous micro-immunotherapeutic preparations that can be used based on individual pathogenesis.

What should I do if I have lactose intolerance?

Lactose is present in Micro-Immunotherapy globules. However, since these are taken sublingually, very little of it reaches the intestines. It needs to be determined whether lactose intolerance is genetic or acquired on a case-by-case basis. Acquired intolerance can be managed with Micro-Immunotherapy.

Note by the author: From 2023 and onwards gradually, all the medications from Labo'Life will appear on the market with new packaging and without lactose.

Can Micro-Immunotherapy be taken preventively?

Certain products that bolster the immune system can be taken preventively. The products developed to enhance brain function in older individuals also serve as preventive measures. However, it's not possible to shield oneself from pathogens (viruses, bacteria) or autoimmune diseases through Micro-Immunotherapy.

Literature

- Bauer, Joachim: Das Gedächtnis des Körpers. Piper Verlag, München, 2004
- Daimler, Renate: Basics der systemischen Strukturaufstellungen. Kösel Verlag, München, 2008
- Doerr, H.W., Gerlich, W.H. (Hrsg.): Medizinische Virologie 2. Auflage; Grundlagen, Diagnostik und Therapie virologischer Krankheitsbilder, Thieme Verlag 2010
- Feinstein, D.; Eden, D.; Graig, G.: Klopf die Sorgen weg. Emotionale Befreiung durch EFT und Energetische Psychologie. Rowohlt Verlag, Reinbek, 2007
- Gallo, F.: Handbuch der Energetischen Psychotherapie. VAK Verlags GmbH, Kirchzarten, 2002
- Glady, G. und Reigh, L.: Studie über die Wirkung der spezifischen Mikroimmuntherapie bei Patienten, die an chronischen Erkrankungen in Verbindung mit dem Epstein-Barr-Virus (EBV) leiden. Erfahrungsheilkunde, Heft 5. Haug Verlag, 2005.
- Hahn, H., Burchard, G.-D., Kaufmann, S.H.E., Schulz, Th.F., Suerbaum, S., (Hrsg.): Medizinische Mikrobiologie und Infektiologie. 6. Auflage. Springer Verlag, Heidelberg 2009
- Heine, H.: Lehrbuch der biologischen Medizin. Hippokrates Verlag, Stuttgart, 1991
- Hof, H., Rüdiger Dörries, R.: Duale Reihe: Medizinische Mikrobiologie. 3. Auflage. Thieme Verlag, Stuttgart 2005
- Hopf-Seidel, P.: Krank nach Zeckenstich. Borreliose erkennen und wirksam behandeln. Knaur Verlag, München, 2008
- Hugot J.P.: Crohn's disease: the cold chain hypothesis, http://dx.doi.org/10.1016/S0140-6736(03)15024-6 [abgerufen:6.5.2016]
- Janeway C.; Travers P.; Walport M.; Shlomchik M.: Immunologie. 5. Auflage, Spektrum Akademischer Verlag GmbH, Heidelberg/Berlin, 2002
- Jenaer M.: Micro-Immunothérapie. La méthode. Eigenverlag Institut 3IDI, 2002
- Jenaer M. et al.: Die Mikroimmuntherapie. 7 grundlegende Wirkungsmechanismen. Eigenverlag Institut 3IDI, 2003
- Jenaer M. et al.: La Micro-Immunothérapie au secours de la Gériatrie. Eigenverlag Institut 3IDI, 2005
- Jenaer M. et al. : Micro-Immunothérapie. Action des cytokines. Eigenverlag Institut 3IDI, 2005
- Jenaer M.: Naissance et spécificités de la Micro-Immunothérapie. Eigenverlag Institut 3IDI, 2007
- Jenaer M.: Die Bedeutung der Mikroimmuntherapie in der Onkologie. ProMed Komplementär, Heft 03, Springer Verlag, Heidelberg, 2005
- Johnson A.: Immunologie auf 70 Seiten. Thieme Verlag, Stuttgart, 2001

- Kandal E.: Auf der Suche nach dem Gedächtnis. Die Entstehung einer neuen Wissenschaft des Geistes. Deutsche Übersetzung, Pantheon Verlag, München, 2007
- Kesslering J.: Multiple Sklerose. 4. überarbeitete und erweiterte Auflage, Kohlhammer, Stuttgart; Berlin; Köln, 2004
- Knipe D. M., Howley P.M. et al. (eds.): Fields´ Virology. 4. Auflage, Philadelphia 2001.
- Levi-Montalcini R.; Calissano P.: The nerve-growth factor. Scientific American, 1979; 240(6): 68–77
- Levi-Montalcini R.: Abbi il Coraggio di Consocere. Rizzoli Verlag, Mailand, 2004
- Merkler, Doron: „Viral déjà vu" elicits organ-specific immune disease independent of reactivity to self. Journal of Clinical Investigation, 2006; 116 (5):1254–63
- Modrow S.; Falke D.; Truyen U.: Molekulare Virologie. Eine Einführung für Biologen und Mediziner. 2. Auflage. Spektrum-Lehrbuch, Heidelberg 2002
- Pert C.: Moleküle der Gefühle. Körper, Geist und Emotionen. Deutsche Übersetzung, Rowohlt Verlag, Reinbek, 2001
- Petter B., Vladimir J. et al.: Variation in the Human Immune System Is Largely Driven by Non-Heritable Influences.
- Pischinger A.: Das System der Grundregulation. 8. erweiterte Auflage, Haug Verlag, Stuttgart, 1990
- Revillard JP.: Immunologie. 4e édition, Edition Larcier, Bruxelles, 2001
- Rose LM, Ginsburg AH, Rothstein TL, Ledbetter JA, Clark EA.: Selective loss of a subset of T helper cells in active multiple sclerosis. Proc Natl Acad Sci USA . 1985;82:7389-7393.
- Santi C., Mor C.: Die Mikroimmuntherapie als ergänzende Krebstherapie. Eine Studie mit Metastasen-Patienten. Journal of Tumor Marker Oncology, The International Academy of Tumor Marker Oncology Inc. Publishers, 2003; 18
- Sobel R., Hafler D., Castro E., Morimoto C., Weiner H. The 2H4 (CD45R) antigen is selectively decreased in multiple sclerosis lesions. J Immunol. 1988; 140:2210-2214.
- Sompayrac L.: How the immune system works. 2nd Edition, Blackwell Publishing, Oxford, UK, 2003
- Steere A.C. et al. (1990): Association of chronic Lymearthritis with HLA-DR4 and HLA-DR2 Alleles. N.Engl. J. Med. 323.
- Steere A.C. et al. (2006): Antibiotic-refractory Lyme arthritis is associated with HLA-DR molecules that bind a Borrelia burgdorferi peptide. JEM 203
- Venken K., Hellings N., Broekmans T., Hensen K, Rummens JL, Stinissen P. Natural naive CD4+CD25+CD127low regulatory T cell (Treg) development and function are disturbed in multiple sclerosis patients: recovery of memory Treg homeostasis during disease progression. J Immunology 2008 May 1;180(9):6411-20. Hasselt

University, Biomedisch Onderzoeksinstituut and Transnationale Universiteit Limburg, School of Life Sciences, Diepenbeek, Belgium.

- Vester F.: Die Kunst, vernetzt zu denken. Ideen und Werkzeuge für einen neuen Umgang mit Komplexität. DVA Verlag, Stuttgart, 2000
- Vester, F.: Leitmotiv vernetztes Denken. Für einen besseren Umgang mit der Welt. Wilhelm Heyne Verlag, München, 1997
- Wang H-L et al: Prevalence of Toxoplasma infection in first-episode schizophrenia and comparison between Toxoplasma-seropositive and Toxoplasma-seronegative schizophrenia. Acta Psychiatrica Scandinavica 2006; 114: 40-48
- Waßmuth R.: Einführung in das HLA-System. Eigenverlag Laborärztliche Arbeitsgemeinschaft für Diagnostik und Rationalisierung e.V., Geesthacht, 2005
- Zinkernagel R.: On reactivity versus tolerance. Immunology and Cell Biology (2004) 82, 343–352; doi:10.1111/j.0818-9641.2004.01255.x

About the Author

- Corinne I. Heitz, PhD 1956 born in Zurich.
- 1975 Graduation High school Zurich
- 1981 Master's degree (lic. phil. I), University of Zurich
- 1983 almost a year's journey by motorbike through India
- since 1987 self-employed in Germany IT and conception, freelancer for General Management of Union Bank of Switzerland
- From 1992 Training as Naturopathic practitioner
- 1995 Examination for cantonally approved alternative practitioner/ ND of the Canton of Appenzell Ausserrhoden (CH)
- 1996 State examination as Heilpraktiker in Tübingen (D)
- May 1996 - April 1997 own practice in Germany
- 1996 - 97 Training in chiropractic according to Dr. Ackermann, Stockholm
- since May 1997 until today practice in Switzerland in 9427 Wolfhalden
- 2000 Lectures on complementary cancer therapies, holistic models in theory and practice, Cusanus Academy, Brixen/Bressanone Italy
- 2001 Diploma in Computer-Regulation-Thermography IMAT
- 2001 Lecture on breast cancer, Cusanus Academy, Brixen/Bressanone Italy
- 2001 Nutrition and Supplements, IEG Richterswil
- 2001 Further training in the field of phytotherapy, especially "hormonal substitution", Gesundheitszentrum GmbH, D-Markdorf
- 2001 - 2002 Western Phytotherapy, HJS-Education
- 2002 Diploma in Homotoxicology (Homotoxicological Society D- Baden-Baden and Albuquerque NM USA)
- from 2002 Courses in "Micro-Immunotherapy" (DeGeMIT/German Society for Micro-Immunotherapy, D-Freiburg)
- 2003 giving courses in computer-regulation thermography
- From 2006 to 2013 President of the "Swiss Association for Micro-Immunotherapy" and trainer for Micro-Immunotherapy (Switzerland)
- 2011 Publication of the book "Mikroimmuntherapie, Diagnostik und Therapie immunologischer Erkrankungen", Foitzick Verlag (today: ML-Verlag), Augsburg 2011
- 2012 Doctorate, University of Zurich Faculty of Philosophy I, PhD with the dissertation "Der Begriff der Gesundheit" (The Term of Health) (interdisciplinary work in philosophy and medicine).
- 2012 Foundation of own publishing house Zwei-Wölfe Verlag GmbH
- 2015 Publication: Die Schilddrüse, Funktion, Erkrankungen, Diagnostik und alternativ-medizinische Therapie, Zwei-Wölfe-Verlag

- 2016 Publication 2nd edition Mikroimmuntherapie (German)
- 2017 Head of department and editor "Health and Diseases" at a health online portal (the project was abandoned)
- 2018 Foundation of https://Naturheilkunde-Akademie.com
- WELL-AGING, SALUTOGENESIS AND MICROIMMUNOTHERAPY
- Colloquium of the Micro-Immunotherapy Platform
- Lochau am Bodensee - 14 to 16 September 2018 Lecture on stress
- 2019 Seminar in Heiden AR July and October
- October 2019 Further training at the BIGmed Congress in A-Krems
- November 2019 Lecture "Concept of Health" at the Salutogenesis Congress of GAMED in Vienna
- Since January 2020 various online seminars at Naturheilkunde-Akademie.com
- Various professional articles and lectures in the context of professional activity.
- 2021 Mikroimmuntherapie, 3rd edition, Mediengruppe Oberfranken
- 2023 Praxisbuch Mikroimmuntherapie 1st edition,

Bibliography

- Mikroimmuntherapie, Foitzick, Augsburg 2011, ISBN 978-3929338560
- Der Begriff der Gesundheit, Zwei-Wölfe Verlag, CH-Wolfhalden 2014, ISBN 978-3906279008
- Die Schilddrüse, Funktion, Erkrankungen, Diagnostik und alternativ-medizinische Therapie, Zwei-Wölfe-Verlag, CH-Wolfhalden, 2015, ISBN 978-3906279015
- Mikroimmuntherapie, 2. Auflage, mgo fachverlage GmbH & Co. KG, Kulmbach; (2017), ISBN: 978-3945695005
- Mikroimmuntherapie, 3. Auflage, mgo fachverlage GmbH & Co. KG, Kulmbach; (2021), ISBN 978-3-96474-503-3
- Praxisbuch Mikroimmuntherapie 1st edition, mgo fachverlage GmbH & Co. KG, Kulmbach; (2023), ISBN: 978-3-96474-243-8

Addresses

Address of the Author

Serafin Naturheilpraxis AG
Corinne I. Heitz, PhD
Kronenstraße 745
9427 Wolfhalden
Switzerland
https://serafin.ch

Training Offered by the Author

The author regularly organises training and further education, information about which can be found on the website: Naturheilkunde-Akademie.com

Reference Laboratories

Specific laboratory tests such as lymphocyte typing, protein profiling and serologies to determine the immune status are carried out in these laboratories:

LADR GmbH
Baden-Baden Medical Care Centre
Contact: Dr. Schüssler
Lange Straße 65
76530 Baden-Baden
Germany
Tel.: +49 (0) 7221 2117-0
Fax: +49 (0) 7221 2117-77
www.ladr.de

Lab4more
Dipl. Biol. Wolfgang Mayer
Augustenstr. 10
80333 Munich
Germany
Customer service: +49 (0) 89 543217-0
Tel.: +49 (0) 89 5432177-89
Fax: +49 (0) 89 5432177-92
wm@immumed.de
www.lab4more-online.de

Medical Diagnostic Laboratory Dr. Dostal
Elisabeth Dostal, MD
Saarplatz 9
1190 Vienna
Austria
Tel.: +43 (0) 1 3683448
Fax: +43 (0) 1 3691269
office@labor-dostal.at
www.labor-dostal.at

Labor Viollier AG
Hagmattstrasse 14
4123 Allschwil
Switzerland
Tel.: +41 (0) 61 4861111
Fax: +41 (0) 61 4820030
contact@viollier.ch
www.viollier.ch

MVZ Labor Dr. Reising-Ackermann and Colleagues
Strümpellstraße 40
04289 Leipzig
Germany
Tel.: +49 (0) 341 6565 - 100
Fax: +49 (0) 341 6565 - 400
info@labor-leipzig.de
www.labor-leipzig.de

Biovis Diagnostik MVZ GmbH
Brüsseler Str. 18
65552 Limburg-Eschhofen
Germany
Tel.: +49 (0) 6431 21248 0
Fax: +49 (0) 6431 21248 66
info@biovis.de
www.biovis.eu

Medical Associations for Micro-Immunotherapy

MeGeMIT – Medizinische Gesellschaft für Mikroimmuntherapie (German speaking Countries)
SPACES/Gertrude-Fröhlich-Sandner-Str. 2, Tower 9
1100 Wien
Austria
Tel.: +43 (0) 1 3027 3040
info@megemit.org
www.MeGeMIT.org

International Website in English

https://www.micro-immunotherapy.com/

French Association

Institut Français de Micro-Immunothérapie
49, rue de Ponthieu
75008 Paris (France)

Spanish Association

Asociación Española de Microinmunoterapia
Av. Portal de l'Àngel, 36
08002 Barcelona (Spain)

Sources of Micro-Immunotherapy, Single Remedies and HLA-SMM

Labo'life Belgium
Parc scientifique CREALYS
11, Rue Camille Hubert
5032 Gembloux
Belgique
https://LaboLife.com

Biomedico, Dublin
Unit 1205, Nesta Storage
4-5 Burton Hall Road
Sandyford
Dublin 18
Ireland
sales@biomedico.ie
www.biomedico.ie

Löwen Apotheke 24
Sandra Hoff, Pharmacist
Lichtentaler Str. 3
76530 Baden-Baden
Germany
info@loewen-apotheke24.de
www.loewen-apotheke24.de

Apotheke zur Kaiserkrone
Mariahilfer Str. 110
1070 Vienna
Austria

Hildegard Pharmacy (Pharmacie)
Rue Auguste De Boeckstraat 45
1140 Brussels
Belgium

Purchase of Preparations from Labo' Life

EU

Labo'Life products are available in all pharmacies within the EU in almost all countries without prescription.

Switzerland

In Switzerland, the products are not registered with Swissmedic and can therefore only be imported and traded under Art. 37 of the Therapeutic Products Act. With a doctor's prescription, pharmacies and self-dispensing doctors can order the products from

Galexis AG
Industriestrasse 2, P.O. Box, 4704 Niederbipp
Tel.: +41 58 851 71 11, Fax: +41 58 851 71 14

Alternative practitioners must provide evidence of their authorization to dispense medications in their practice.

Patients in Switzerland can visit any pharmacy with a prescription from a doctor.

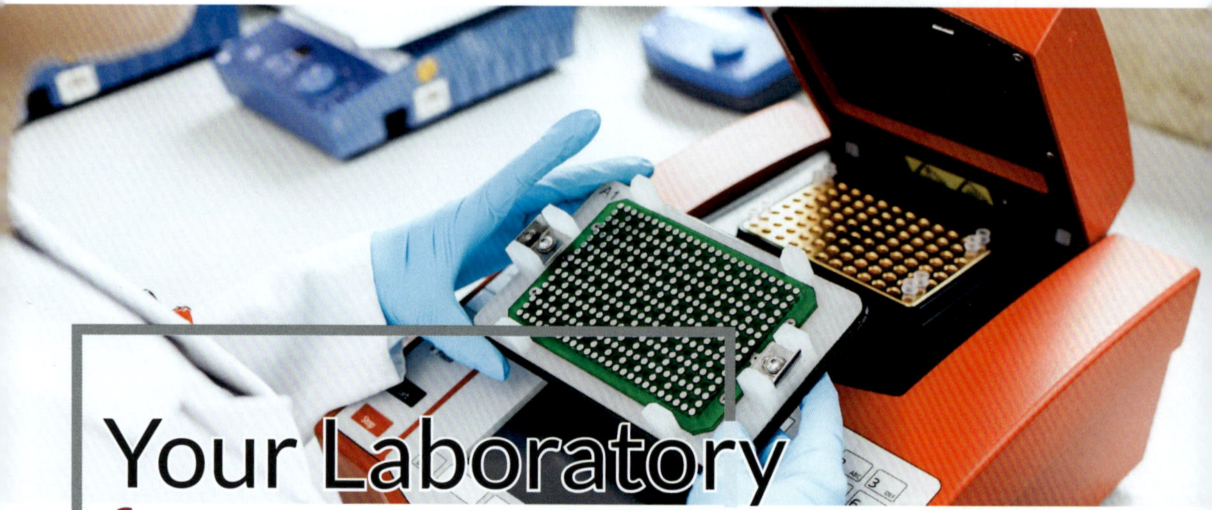

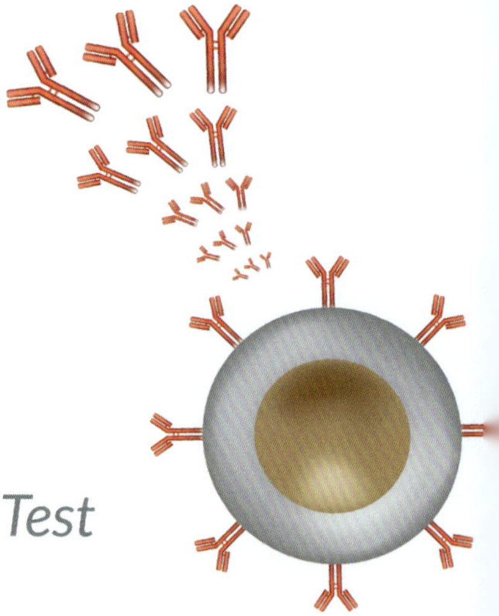